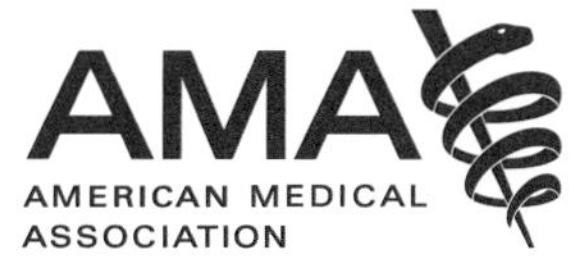

E/M Office Visit Compendium 2021

Resources for understanding changes to CPT® coding for office visits

Executive Vice President, Chief Executive Officer: James L. Madara, MD
Senior Vice President, Health Solutions: Laurie A.S. McGraw
Vice President, Coding and Reimbursement Policy and Strategy: Jay Ahlman
Director, CPT Coding and Regulatory Services: Zach Hochstetler
Director, CPT Content Management & Development: Leslie W. Prellwitz
Manager, CPT Content Management and Development: Karen E. O'Hara
CPT Senior Healthcare Coding Analyst: Janette Meggs
CPT Senior Healthcare Coding Analyst: Donna Tyler
Senior Healthcare Coding Analyst: Arletrice Watkins
CPT Healthcare Coding Analyst: Andrei Besleaga
CPT Healthcare Coding Analyst: Rejina Young
Vice President, Operations: Denise C. Foy
Publishing Operations Manager: Elizabeth Goodman Duke
Senior Developmental Editor: Lisa Chin-Johnson
Production Specialist: Mary Ann Albanese
Vice President, Sales: Lori Prestesater
Director, Channel Sales: Erin Kalitowski
Executive, Key Account Manager: Mark Daniels
Vice President, Product Management: Dave Sosnow
Director, CPT Operations & Infrastructure: Barbara Benstead
Product Manager, Print and Digital Products: Mark Ruthman
Marketing Manager: Vanessa Prieto

Printed in the United States of America. 20 21 22/ TB-WC / 9 8 7 6 5 4 3 2 1

ISBN: 978-1-64016-042-2

To purchase additional CPT products, contact the American Medical Association Customer Service at 800 621-8335 or visit the AMA|Store at **amastore.com**.

Refer to product number OP504021.

To request a license for distribution of products containing or reprinting CPT codes and/or guidelines, please see our website at www.ama-assn.org/go/cpt, or contact the American Medical Association CPT/DBP Intellectual Property Services, 330 North Wabash Avenue, Suite 39300, Chicago, IL 60611, 312 464-5022.

AC30:OP504021:11/20

Contents

Section 2: E/M 2021: MDM and Code-Level Selection Changes

Section 3: E/M 2021: Time and Code-Level Selection Changes

Using The Book

The *E/M Office Visit Compendium 2021* is intended as a supplement to the Current Procedural Terminology (CPT®) 2021 codebook, providing helpful context and detailed explanations for the E/M office visit code revisions. The resources in this book will help coders, billers, and educators understand how to apply the revised office visit codes, the shorter prolonged services codes, and the revised criteria for leveling. For more information on related non-E/M codes, see the *CPT® Professional 2021* codebook.

The resources in this book are designed with the intermediate user in mind. Those who are unfamiliar with the fundamentals of E/M coding, or CPT codes more generally, may find it useful to begin with *Principles of CPT® Coding*, a comprehensive introduction to CPT billing and coding guidelines.

The revision of codes and coding guidelines for outpatient evaluation and management (E/M) services (99202-99215) in CPT 2021 represents the first major overhaul of E/M reporting in more than 25 years. These changes have the potential to give physicians and other qualified health care professionals (QHPs) more time to spend with patients by freeing them from significant administrative burden.

The revisions can be summarized as follows:

- **History and physical examination have been eliminated as elements for code selection.**
    - History and physical examination should not determine the appropriate code level selected. While the physician's or other QHP's work in capturing the patient's pertinent history and performing a relevant physical examination contributes to both the time and the medical decision making (MDM) involved in the encounter, these elements alone should not determine the appropriate code level.
    - Health care professionals should perform a medically appropriate history and/or examination.
- **The physician or other QHP is allowed to choose whether to base the documentation on MDM or on total time:**
    - The MDM definitions have been revised and clarified.
    - The definition of time has been revised to specify ranges instead of a typical time and to represent total physician/QHP time on the date of service. The definition of time applies only when code selection is based primarily on time and not when it is based on MDM.
- **Code 99201 has been deleted.**
    - Code 99201 has been deleted because codes 99201 and 99202 had straightforward MDM.
- **A shorter prolonged services code has been created.**
    - A shorter prolonged services code (99417), which captures physician/QHP time in 15-minute increments, has been created.
    - This code should be reported only with codes 99205 and 99215 when time is the primary basis for code selection.

Keep in mind that these changes apply only to office and other outpatient services (99202-99215).

The first chapter provides a summary of the changes in the guideline structure to show readers the changes. In addition, a summary of the changes is available in Appendix A to provide information on the changes in the guidelines to assist readers in understanding where sections of the the guidelines may have been relocated for the CPT 2021 code set.

The most effective way to use this book is to:

- Review the CPT code descriptors and guidelines for 2021 E/M office visit codes.
- Examine the new summary of changes table in this book.
    - The table illustrates the differences between the 2020 and 2021 E/M office or other outpatient codes.
    - Understanding and use of this table will assist in accurate E/M code selection.

- Inspect the updated MDM table included in this book.
  - Review the updated and new definitions for clarity.
  - Familiarize yourself with this table to assist in appropriate 2021 E/M code selection.
- Analyze the updates for reporting time under the 2021 guidelines.
  - In 2021, if code selection for office or other outpatient services is based on time, the time will be the total time on the date of the encounter as opposed to face-to-face time during the encounter.
- Verify the guidelines for using the new prolonged services code before reporting.
  - Code 99417 may be reported only with codes 99205 and 99215 when the code selection is primarily based on time.
  - When the new prolonged services code is reported, the prolonged service time starts at the minimum total time for codes 99205 and 99215. As an example, for a new patient encounter (99205), 60 minutes of time are required to report the service. Do not report code 99417 until at least 15 minutes of time has been accumulated beyond the required 60 minutes (ie, 75 minutes) on the date of the encounter.
- Assess the pending changes.
  - Evaluate your current E/M office visit usage and patterns.
    - Review internal systems or practices that will need to be revised to accommodate the deletion of code 99201.
    - Confirm that your electronic health record vendor is on target with updates for your system(s).
- Review current time-based vs MDM-based code selection for its impact on your practice.
  - Determine, based on your assessment of the changes and specific patient circumstances, when to choose MDM vs total time documented for visit.
  - Adjust practice policies for more efficient use of resources based on the new guidelines.
- Explore the new E/M guidelines to understand the criteria to be used when selecting other types of E/M codes.
  - The changes for 2021 focus on the office or other outpatient codes (99202-99215) and the related prolonged services code (99417).
  - Other E/M codes (eg, hospital observation, hospital inpatient, consultations, emergency department, critical care, nursing facility and domiciliary, rest home services) will continue to use the current existing criteria and definitions for selection.

About CPT

Current Procedural Terminology (CPT®), Fourth Edition, is a listing of descriptive terms and identifying codes for reporting medical services and procedures performed by physicians and other qualified health care professionals. It provides a uniform language that accurately describes medical, surgical, and diagnostic services, and thereby provides an effective means for reliable nationwide communication among physicians and other qualified health care professionals, patients, and third parties. CPT 2021 is the most recent revision of a work that first appeared in 1966.

CPT descriptive terms and identifying codes currently serve a wide variety of important functions in the field of medical nomenclature. The CPT code set is useful for administrative management purposes such as claims processing and for the development of guidelines for medical care review. The uniform language is also applicable to medical education and outcomes, health services, and quality research by providing a useful basis for local, regional, and national utilization comparisons. The CPT code set is the most widely accepted nomenclature for the reporting of physician and other qualified health care professional procedures and services under government and private health insurance programs. In 2000, the CPT code set was designated by the Department of Health and Human Services as the national coding standard for physician and other health care professional services and procedures under the Health Insurance Portability and Accountability Act (HIPAA). This means that for all financial and administrative health care transactions sent electronically, the CPT code set will need to be used.

The changes outlined in this book have been prepared by the CPT Editorial Panel with the assistance of physicians and representatives of other health care professions representing all specialties of medicine, and with important contributions from many third-party payers and governmental agencies. E/M office visit codes are used to report evaluation and management services provided in the office or in an outpatient or other ambulatory facility, and the American Medical Association trusts that this supplemental publication will extend the usefulness of CPT 2021 and other CPT publications in identifying, describing, and coding medical, surgical, and diagnostic services.

Current CPT Editorial Panel

The Symbols

This book uses the same code symbol conventions as those used in the CPT code set.

- ● Indicates a new procedure number was added to the CPT nomenclature
- ▲ Indicates a code revision has resulted in a substantially altered procedure descriptor
- ✚ Indicates a CPT add-on code
- ⊘ Indicates a code that is exempt from the use of modifier 51 but is not designated as a CPT add-on procedure or service
- ▶◀ Indicates revised guidelines, cross-references, and/or explanatory text
- ⚡ Indicates a code for a vaccine that is pending FDA approval
- # Indicates a resequenced code. Note that rather than deleting and renumbering, resequencing allows existing codes to be relocated to an appropriate location for the code concept, regardless of the numeric sequence. Numerically placed references (ie, Code is out of numerical sequence. See . . .) are used as navigational alerts in the CPT codebook to direct the user to the location of an out-of-sequence code. Therefore, remember to refer to the CPT codebook for these references.
- ★ Indicates a telemedicine code
- ♓ Indicates a duplicate PLA test
- ⇅ Indicates a Category I PLA test

Preface

The *E/M Office Visit Compendium 2021* is the result of a kernel of thought generated back in 2018, after the need for changes in some of the evaluation and management (E/M) codes in the Current Procedural Terminology (CPT®) code set had been recognized but before the CPT Editorial Panel had voted to implement the changes.

From one perspective, these changes were no more than a routine code-change proposal to be voted on at an upcoming CPT Editorial Panel meeting, with the usual required preparation and deadlines. A total of 11 codes, barely one-tenth of 1% of the entire CPT code set, would be involved. The proposal would include revisions to nine existing codes, the deletion of one code, and the addition of one new code, along with language revisions in the associated guidelines. By that measure, it was an ordinary, revision: other code-change proposals have certainly involved more than 11 codes in total and more than 10 existing codes.

From another perspective, the change was anything but routine. These 10 codes are used by physicians and other health care professionals in nearly every specialty for the reporting of office and other outpatient visits. These codes account for roughly 25% of total spending for physician services under Medicare Part B and have a similar impact on non-Medicare payments. Given their extremely widespread use and economic impact in the industry, even the slightest change in these codes would result in a wave of impact, requiring an extraordinary level of coordination across specialty societies for success.

These 10 codes involve some of the most complex reporting guidelines and processes to select the appropriate code for a given service. Many coders will clearly remember the journeys they took to learn the first set of guidelines in 1995 and to expand their learning with the 1997 release. The tables, the definitions, the assessment of the level of history and examination, and the identification of the rubrics of "two of three" key components, all served to form the basis of a common language across the individuals who used the codes to report services and the computerized billing and audit systems that analyzed claims data. Over more than a quarter century, that language has become established and ingrained in individuals' minds and in computer logic.

Given the broad impact of these changes, the American Medical Association (AMA) embarked on an unprecedented initiative to provide early notification to prepare the industry for a smooth transition. The AMA recognized that the coding community and all who use the CPT code set needed to have sufficient lead time to absorb this new E/M dialect, a change similar to the transition from ICD-9-CM to ICD-10-CM.

Along with the need for early notification, it was foreseen that there would be a need to ensure that the most salient changes, impacts, and learning aids were clearly and readily accessible, in one location, to both current and upcoming CPT code users so that they would have all the information at their fingertips when it is needed. With that foresight, the *E/M Office Visit Compendium 2021* idea was launched.

Cognizant of the fact that the E/M changes for 2021 affect only a subset of E/M codes, this book is designed to focus on those specific changes, so as not to detract from the significant investment the reader has already made in learning the E/M guidelines and practices that have not been affected.

The book is divided into six sections. The first section provides a background on the genesis of the changes and the early efforts of the Centers for Medicare & Medicaid Services (CMS) and the AMA, including the goals and principles of the CPT/RUC Workgroup on E/M and a high-level summary of the changes. Subsequent sections provide additional information and insight on each of the main change categories. Section 2 outlines the substantial changes made in medical decision making (MDM), while Sections 3 and 4 focus on time and the new prolonged services code, respectively. Section 5 presents the E/M guidelines and codes from the *CPT® Professional 2021* codebook. Section 6 includes a tabular summary of guideline changes for the entire E/M section and other useful resources.

The structure of the book was set up so that the materials could be quickly absorbed by those who are actively coding in a busy practice environment, with little time to review the changes in advance of their effective date in January 2021. In 2018 and 2019, it was believed that the majority of health care professionals would have ample time in 2020 to review and incorporate the needed changes in their practices and workflows. At the time, no one could have foreseen the emergence of a certain coronavirus and the resulting stresses and strains placed on the health care system during the COVID-19 pandemic. The AMA hopes that this book will serve as a useful resource to all who need to understand and incorporate the 2021 E/M changes.

Introduction

Physicians and other qualified health care professionals (QHPs) know that the time required to document patient encounters often results in reduced time for patient care and more time spent completing medical records. For several decades, electronic health records (EHRs) have required standardized documentation for each encounter, which has led to a systemic issue: note bloat. Note bloat, or excessive copying and pasting of data between sections of the medical record in an effort to meet documentation requirements, results in the meaningless accumulation of data, often not pertinent to the reason for the encounter. This extensive, confusing documentation takes additional time to produce and review, leading to increased time outside clinic hours. A study published in *Annals of Internal Medicine* in 2016 documented that, for every hour physicians spent performing direct patient care, they spent nearly two additional hours performing administrative and EHR work. In addition, each day ended with another one to two hours of administrative work at home.[1] These hours, which often go unpaid, are a contributing factor in the increased physician burnout rates seen over the past decade. Ultimately, unnecessary documentation leads to physician burnout and to patient records that are less clinically relevant and difficult to navigate, which can have numerous consequences for patient care.

Revising the evaluation and management (E/M) documentation guidelines for office or other outpatient services (99201-99215) for the Current Procedural Terminology (CPT®) 2021 code set represented a perfect opportunity to address these systemic issues. The CPT Editorial Panel had previously identified this series of codes as a key issue for modification in 2012, when large-scale revisions were approved but never published. In summer 2018, the completion of this seismic change was galvanized when the Centers for Medicare & Medicaid Services (CMS) released the Medicare physician fee schedule proposed rule for calendar year 2019. This rule outlined several large initiatives dedicated to simplifying documentation requirements for office E/M visits. Many of these initiatives were aimed in the right direction, but they only addressed symptoms of the underlying issue: the documentation requirements themselves. The documentation standards needed to be revised and standardized into a single set of guidelines that would be incorporated into the CPT code set for use by Medicare and Medicaid and commercial payers across the country.

Over a six-month period, a dedicated and committed workgroup of clinical experts convened by the American Medical Association (AMA), including physicians and other QHPs, sought input from hundreds of additional experts from all sectors of health care to revise the documentation guidelines for office or other outpatient E/M visits. At each step of the way, the CPT and AMA/Specialty Society Relative Value Scale (RVS) Update Committee (RUC) E/M Workgroup sought consensus and real-world experience to inform the revisions. A clear set of four guiding principles enabled the workgroup to target the revisions directly to meet the objectives.

Principle 1: Decrease administrative burden of documentation and coding

The workgroup addressed this principle by removing the mandatory history and physical examination elements. The revised system focuses the code selection on how physicians and other QHPs use their cognitive skills to diagnose and manage the patient's condition.

Principle 2: Decrease the need for audits via the addition and expansion of key definitions and guidelines

The workgroup addressed this principle by providing additional, extensive detail in the CPT guidelines, outlining key definitions that had been the source of confusion for decades. This level of detail was intended to promote not only consistency of coding but also consistency in audits, if performed.

Principle 3: Decrease unnecessary documentation in the medical record that is not needed for patient care

This principle was addressed by eliminating code-level selection based on a count of bulleted items related to the history and physical examination. The workgroup also sought to support the importance and value of higher-level activities of medical decision making (MDM). This meant shifting the focus from items such as the number of elements examined in a review of systems to higher-level activities such as assessing the complexity of the patient's problems, analyzing complex data, and sharing decision making with other clinicians in the collaborative management of patients with multiple conditions.

Principle 4: Ensure that payment for E/M services is resource-based and has no direct goal of payment redistribution among specialties

This objective was achieved by using the current MDM criteria, along with current Medicare and commercial payer educational and audit tools, to form the basis of the revised MDM code-selection criteria. By maintaining consistency with existing structures, this process reduced the likelihood of large shifts in coding practices across different specialties.

As with any change, it will take time for stakeholders to fully adapt to the new changes. However, the simplified E/M office visit reporting guidelines represent significant improvements. The revisions approved by the CPT Editorial Panel for 2021 offer the potential for a future in which documentation is less burdensome and patient care is improved.

The process involved seeking input from many stakeholders. It is necessary to thank the workgroup, all the specialty society advisors and staff, coding professionals, and the dedicated and resourceful AMA staff. Finally, great appreciation is expressed to the CMS administrator for leadership and commitment in helping to reduce administrative burden and for the collaboration with CMS personnel that helped to ensure acceptance of the revisions and smooth progress through the rule-making process.

Reference

1. Sinsky C, Colligan L, Li L, et al. Allocation of physician time in ambulatory practice: A time and motion study in 4 specialties. *Ann Intern Med.* 2016;165(11):753-760. doi:10.7326/M16-0961.

Acknowledgments

This book represents the cumulative efforts of many individuals across the AMA and CPT spectrum, too numerous to list individually. The AMA would like to acknowledge and thank everyone for their efforts over the past years, particularly the following groups:

AMA CPT staff
AMA RUC staff
CPT Editorial Panel
CPT/RUC Workgroup on E/M
CPT® Assistant Editorial Board

A special mention and thanks to Peter Hollmann, MD, and Barbara Levy, MD, co-chairs of the E/M workgroup, for their leadership and guidance on this initiative, to Patrick Carey, for his steadfast assistance in the writing and organization of the manuscript, and to CPT staff members Jennifer Bell, BS, RHIT, CPC, CPMA, CPC-I, CEMC, CPEDC, and Lianne Stancik, BA, RHIT, for their unwavering efforts to manage all the details of the E/M proposals and changes, and for providing invaluable feedback on the materials used to prepare this book.

SECTION 1
Setting the Foundation

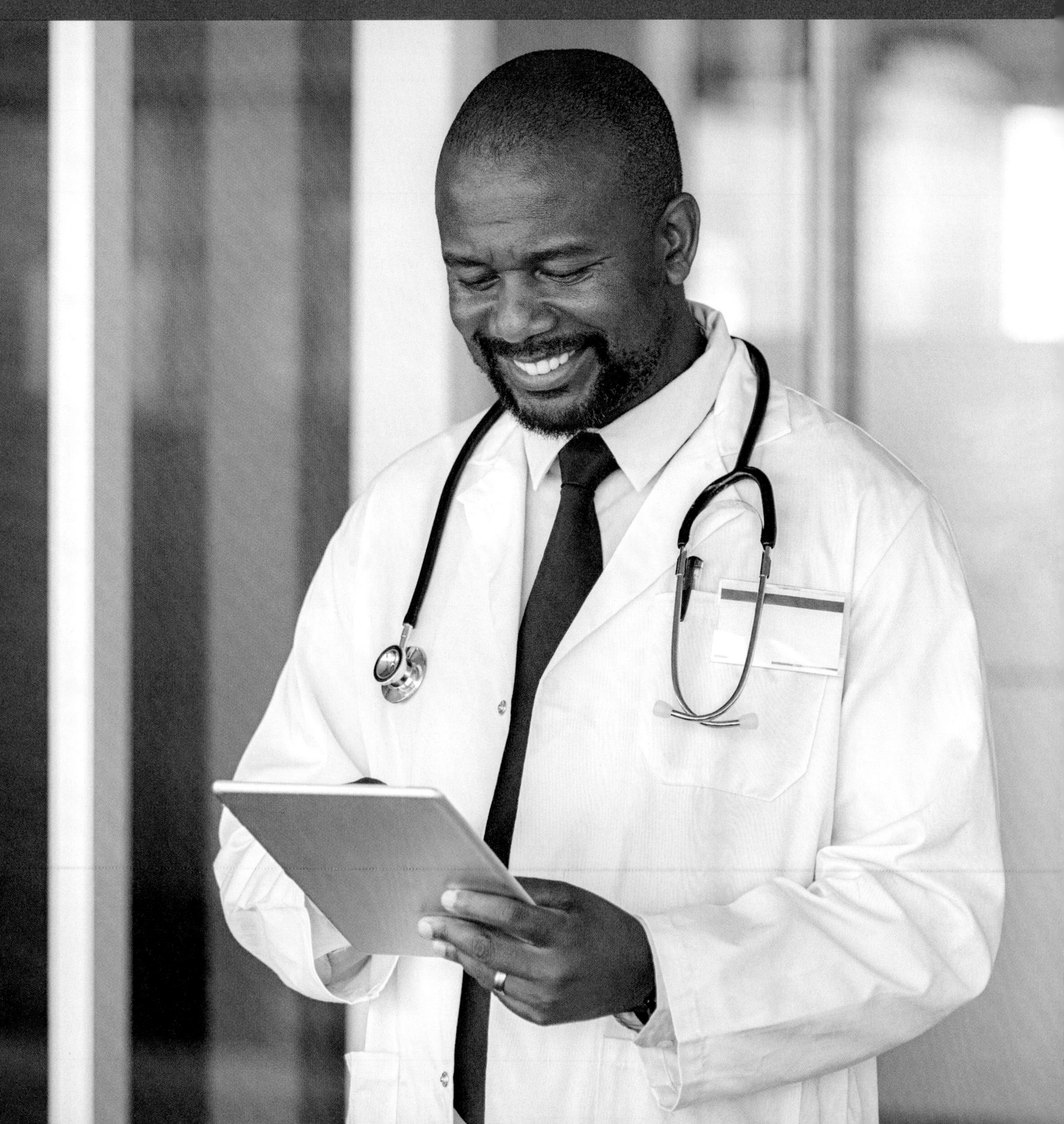

This section offers a grounded view of the background and history of the evaluation and management (E/M) office or other outpatient visit code revisions effective January 1, 2021. From the initial proposal for E/M code changes by the Centers for Medicare & Medicaid Services (CMS) through the efforts of the American Medical Association (AMA) E/M Workgroup and the resulting coding and guideline changes, this section provides key insights on how the 2021 changes came about. This section also summarizes the revisions. As a quick reference, it will be helpful to anyone working with new patient, established patient, prolonged service, and other codes.

The objectives of this section are as follows:

- Understand the initial drivers of the E/M code changes
- Learn about the AMA E/M Workgroup
- Get a quick overview of the key revisions of the E/M codes for the Current Procedural Terminology (CPT®) 2021 code set

CHAPTER 1

Background and Revision Summary

Background: Rationale and Goals for Change

Some fundamental background of the rationale and goals of the changes in the 2021 evaluation and management (E/M) codes for office or other outpatient visits will provide a more complete perspective and understanding of the following changes discussed in this chapter.

Catalyst for Change: Medicare 2019 Fee Schedule

Although revisions to the E/M codes for office or other outpatient visits had been debated for years, the road to the 2021 E/M changes in the Current Procedural Terminology (CPT®) 2021 code set began in earnest in July 2018, with the release of the Medicare Physician Payment Schedule proposed rule for calendar year 2019. In that rule, CMS proposed major initiatives to revise the documentation requirements and payment levels for office or other outpatient visit E/M codes. The revisions were part of CMS' broader "Patients over Paperwork" initiative, which included administrative simplification as a key goal.

The main tenets of the proposed rule included:

- Elimination of the requirement to document the medical necessity of conducting visits in the home rather than in the office.
- Elimination of the prohibition on same-day E/M visits billed by physicians or other qualified health care professionals (QHPs) in the same group or medical specialty.
- Ability of physicians or other QHPs to choose their method of documentation, using the CMS 1995/1997 guidelines, medical decision making (MDM) only, or face-to-face time.
- Elimination of reentry of information regarding chief complaint and history already recorded by ancillary staff or the patient. The physician or other QHP must only document that they reviewed and verified the information.
- Condensed payment amounts for Level 2 through 5 visits, along with offsets for selected specialties through the use of an additional code.
- Elimination of payment for E/M and procedures provided on the same day.

Proposed rule
The official document that announces and explains a federal agency's plan to address a problem or accomplish a goal. All proposed rules must be published in the *Federal Register* to notify the public and give the public an opportunity to submit comments. The proposed rule and the public comments received on it form the basis of the final rule.

Physician or other qualified health care professional (QHP)
An individual who is qualified by education, training, licensure/regulation (when applicable), and facility privileging (when applicable) who performs a professional service within the individual's scope of practice and independently reports that professional service.

To respond appropriately to the variety of coding and reimbursement changes proposed by CMS, a coordinated effort to obtain and gather input from a wide range of specialties was essential to ensure that all viewpoints were considered and incorporated.

The Response: E/M Workgroup

In response to the proposed rule, the AMA convened the CPT and AMA/Specialty Society Relative Value Scale (RVS) Update Committee (RUC) E/M Workgroup. The workgroup was tasked with proposing a comprehensive set of recommendations based on input from a diverse group of clinical experts, including the national medical specialty societies, commercial payer representatives, and CMS policy officials.

With a focus on transparency and inclusion, the workgroup conducted a number of activities to obtain suggestions and feedback. A series of seven open calls as well as a face-to-face meeting were held to address the tenets necessary to adequately modernize the E/M reporting guidelines and reduce their administrative burden. The calls involved, on average, over 200 participants each and included not only representatives of specialty societies but also commercial and government payers as well as CMS staff. The proposal also garnered the attention of a significant number of interested parties. A series of five targeted surveys provided additional insights from nearly 60 stakeholder organizations.

At the same time, the AMA, along with 170 organizations, encompassing medical specialty societies and 50 state medical associations, submitted a letter to CMS. This letter addressed three areas of consensus and concern. The first area provided consensus recommendations for streamlining documentation requirements by only requiring documentation of patient history that had changed in the interval since the previous visit, eliminating the requirement to redocument information already collected by practice staff or patients, and removing the need to justify home visits in place of office visits. The second area was a concern regarding the potential unintended consequences of payment-rate consolidation across service levels, including disproportionate adverse effects on certain specialties that provide complex care. Similarly, the third area provided feedback on the unintended consequences of reducing payment for office visits occurring on the same day as other services.

Throughout the summer of 2018, the workgroup continued its efforts to delineate how the CPT code descriptors and guidelines would need to be adjusted to achieve the overarching goal of reducing the administrative burden and simplifying documentation for health care professionals, while maintaining four guiding principles of resource-based care (Table 1).

Relative Value Scale (RVS) Update Committee (RUC)
An expert panel of physicians that makes recommendations to the government on the resources required to provide a medical service. The expert panel's assessment takes into account physicians' time, nurses' time, and the supplies and equipment involved in patient care. RUC consists of a volunteer group of 31 physicians and 300 medical advisors that represent each sector of medicine, including primary care physicians and specialists. RUC regularly reviews medical services to determine whether they are appropriately valued, undervalued, or overvalued and provides its recommendations to CMS for the agency's consideration. CMS makes all final decisions about payments for each service under the Medicare program.

TABLE 1 The E/M Workgroup's Four Guiding Principles of Resource-Based Care

Principle 1	Decrease administrative burden of documentation and coding
Principle 2	Decrease the need for audits via the addition and expansion of key definitions and guidelines
Principle 3	Decrease unnecessary documentation in the medical record that is not needed for patient care
Principle 4	Ensure that payment for E/M services is resource-based and has no direct goal of payment redistribution among specialties

The CPT Editorial Panel ultimately approved the workgroup's recommendations for publication in the CPT 2021 code set. On November 1, 2019, CMS finalized the decision to accept and implement the revisions to the CPT office or other outpatient visit E/M codes. **These changes will go into effect on January 1, 2021.**

Summary of Changes

The key changes in the office or other outpatient visit E/M codes, along with factors considered by the E/M workgroup (where applicable), are summarized below. Each change will be addressed in greater detail in the sections that follow.

- Revisions of the code descriptors for codes 99202-99205 and 99211-99215;
- Addition of a shorter prolonged service code (99417);
- Deletion of code 99201;
- Elimination of history and/or physical examination as a component for code selection;
- Allowing the use of MDM or time for code level selection;
- Changes in the definitions of MDM and time when used to report these codes; and
- Extensive E/M guideline additions, revisions, and restructuring.

Changes to Code Structure

E/M codes typically have a defined and extensive code structure, reflecting the components evaluated in code selection. The basic format of many codes for face-to-face E/M services is as follows (see the schematic diagram of a current E/M office or other outpatient code in Figure 1):

- The place or type of service is specified (eg, office or other outpatient setting).
- The content and extent of the service are defined (eg, a problem-focused history, a problem-focused examination, straightforward MDM).
- Counseling and/or coordination of care with other health care professionals or agencies are included when an E/M service is reported, if appropriate.
- The nature of the presenting problem(s), usually associated with a given level, is described.
- The typical time associated with the provision of the service is noted in many codes.

The revised office or other outpatient visit E/M codes for 2021 have a considerably more streamlined structure, reflecting the decreased documentation burden for code selection (see Figure 2). The requirement of counseling and/or coordination of care has been removed, and the content-of-service area in the code description specifies a medically appropriate history and/or examination, rather than specific levels.

FIGURE 1 Schematic Example of a 2020 E/M Office or Other Outpatient Code

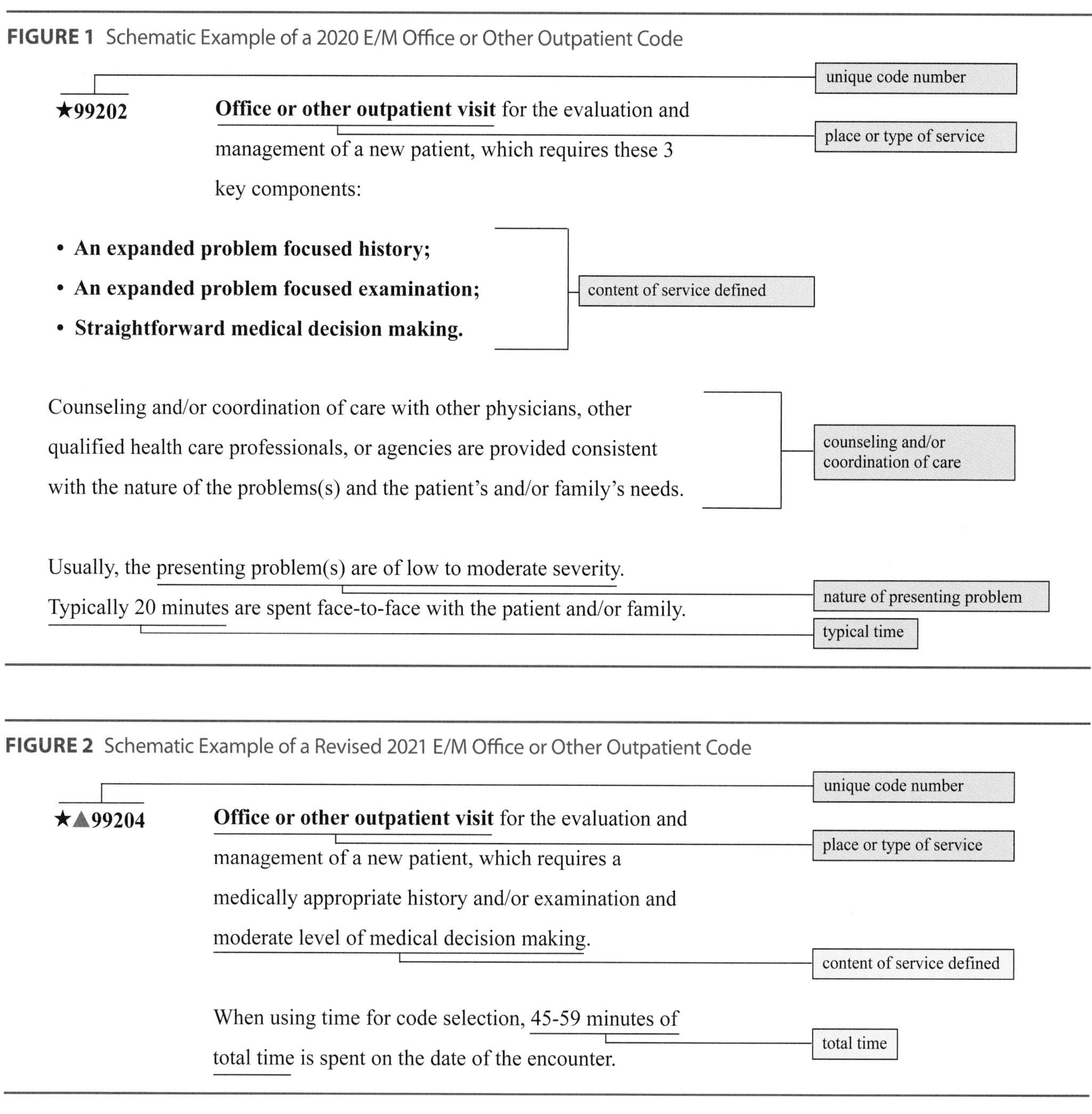

FIGURE 2 Schematic Example of a Revised 2021 E/M Office or Other Outpatient Code

★▲99204 **Office or other outpatient visit** for the evaluation and management of a new patient, which requires a medically appropriate history and/or examination and moderate level of medical decision making.

unique code number

place or type of service

content of service defined

When using time for code selection, 45-59 minutes of total time is spent on the date of the encounter.

total time

Revised Code Descriptors

A list of the revised descriptors for codes 99202-99205 and 99211-99215 is provided below. Users should always consult the CPT 2021 code set for the final approved list of descriptors, parenthetical notes, and associated guidelines.

New Patient

►(99201 has been deleted. To report, use 99202)◄

★▲99202 **Office or other outpatient visit** for the evaluation and management of a new patient, which requires a medically appropriate history and/or examination and straightforward medical decision making.

When using time for code selection, 15-29 minutes of total time is spent on the date of the encounter.

★▲99203 **Office or other outpatient visit** for the evaluation and management of a new patient, which requires a medically appropriate history and/or examination and low level of medical decision making.

When using time for code selection, 30-44 minutes of total time is spent on the date of the encounter.

★▲99204 **Office or other outpatient visit** for the evaluation and management of a new patient, which requires a medically appropriate history and/or examination and moderate level of medical decision making.

When using time for code selection, 45-59 minutes of total time is spent on the date of the encounter.

★▲99205 **Office or other outpatient visit** for the evaluation and management of a new patient, which requires a medically appropriate history and/or examination and high level of medical decision making.

When using time for code selection, 60-74 minutes of total time is spent on the date of the encounter.

►(For services 75 minutes or longer, use prolonged services 99417)◄

Established Patient

▲99211 **Office or other outpatient visit** for the evaluation and management of an established patient, that may not require the presence of a physician or other qualified health care professional. Usually, the presenting problem(s) are minimal.

★▲99212 **Office or other outpatient visit** for the evaluation and management of an established patient, which requires a medically appropriate history and/or examination and straightforward medical decision making.

When using time for code selection, 10-19 minutes of total time is spent on the date of the encounter.

★▲99213 **Office or other outpatient visit** for the evaluation and management of an established patient, which requires a medically appropriate history and/or examination and low level of medical decision making.

When using time for code selection, 20-29 minutes of total time is spent on the date of the encounter.

★▲99214 **Office or other outpatient visit** for the evaluation and management of an established patient, which requires a medically appropriate history and/or examination and moderate level of medical decision making.

When using time for code selection, 30-39 minutes of total time is spent on the date of the encounter.

★▲99215 **Office or other outpatient visit** for the evaluation and management of an established patient, which requires a medically appropriate history and/or examination and high level of medical decision making.

When using time for code selection, 40-54 minutes of total time is spent on the date of the encounter.

▶(For services 55 minutes or longer, use prolonged services 99417)◀

Creation of Shorter Prolonged Service Code

A shorter prolonged service add-on code to report additional physician and/or QHP time in 15-minute increments has been approved for CPT 2021. This five-digit code, 99417, will be reported only with the codes with the longest time ranges (99205 or 99215) and is used only when time is the basis for code selection.

▸Prolonged Service With or Without Direct Patient Contact on the Date of an Office or Other Outpatient Service◂

#★+●99417 Prolonged office or other outpatient evaluation and management service(s) beyond the minimum required time of the primary procedure which has been selected using total time), requiring total time with or without direct patient contact beyond the usual service, on the date of the primary service, each 15 minutes of total time (List separately in addition to codes 99205, 99215 for office or other outpatient **Evaluation and Management** services)

▶(Use 99417 in conjunction with 99205, 99215)◀

▶(Do not report 99417 on the same date of service as 99354, 99355, 99358, 99359, 99415, 99416)◀

▶(Do not report 99417 for any time unit less than 15 minutes)◀

Changes to Code Usage

In the process of formulating the changes, the E/M workgroup and the CPT Editorial Panel considered various aspects of both current and evolving practice patterns to facilitate adoption and appropriate usage of the codes. Some of those considerations are outlined below.

- **Eliminate history and physical examination as elements for code selection:** While the physician's work in capturing the patient's pertinent history and performing a relevant physical examination contributes to both time and MDM, these elements alone should not determine the appropriate code level. Therefore, the workgroup has revised the code descriptors to state that physicians should perform a "medically appropriate history and/or examination."
- **Allow physicians to choose whether their documentation is based on MDM or total time:**
    - **MDM:** The workgroup has not materially changed the three components of MDM, but it has made extensive edits to the elements for code selection and provided numerous clarifying definitions in the E/M guidelines.
    - **Time:** Time is defined as the total time, not typical time, and it represents total physician or other QHP time spent on the date of service. The use of date-of-service time builds on the movement over the last several years by Medicare to better recognize the work involved in services that are not performed face to face, such as care coordination. These definitions apply only when code selection is based primarily on time, *not* when it is based on MDM.
- **Modify the criteria for MDM:** The CPT Editorial Panel used the current CMS Table of Risk as a foundation for revising the elements required for MDM. Current CMS contractor-audit tools were also consulted to minimize disruption in the criteria for MDM levels.
    - Removed ambiguous terms (eg, *mild*) and defined previously ambiguous concepts (eg, *acute or chronic illness with systemic symptoms*).
    - Defined important terms, such as *independent historian*.
    - Redefined the data element to move away from simply adding up tasks, to focus on tasks that affect the management of the patient (eg, independent interpretation of a test performed by another health care professional and/or discussion of test interpretation with an external physician or other QHP).
- **Delete code 99201:** The CPT Editorial Panel agreed to eliminate code 99201 because codes 99201 and 99202 were both straightforward MDM codes that were differentiated only by the history and examination elements.

Changes to Guidelines

Along with the changes to the codes, the E/M guidelines have also undergone revisions, which are outlined here. The two main types of revisions involve (1) use of the new and revised codes and (2) a bifurcation of the E/M guideline structure to accommodate both the revised codes and those that remain unchanged for 2021.

Key Aspects of Guideline Changes for New and Revised E/M Codes

The following are some of the key aspects of the changes in the guidelines for new and revised E/M codes.

Code-Selection Components Streamlined

One of the most significant changes for E/M code selection involves the components used to select the appropriate code for the level of service provided. Prior to 2021, the descriptors of the service levels for office or other outpatient visit E/M codes recognized seven components, six of which could be used in defining the service level:

- History
- Examination
- MDM
- Counseling
- Coordination of care
- Nature of presenting problem
- Time

Before 2021, the first three of these (history, examination, and MDM) were considered key components in selecting the E/M service level; time was the controlling factor only when counseling and/or coordination of care dominated (ie, accounted for > 50% of) the encounter with the patient and/or family. In addition, only face-to-face time on the date of the encounter was to be used in determining the service level for time-based coding of office, outpatient, or ambulatory visits.

Effective January 1, 2021, selection of the appropriate service level for E/M office or other outpatient visit codes will be based on:

- The level of MDM as defined for each service; or
- The total physician or other QHP time for the E/M services on the date of the encounter.

History and physical examination should still be performed and/or documented as medically appropriate, but these elements will no longer be used for code selection. Code 99201 has been deleted from the CPT 2021 code set because codes 99201 and 99202 both had straightforward MDM and were differentiated only by the history and examination elements.

Revisions to Definition of Time

Effective January 1, 2021, time will be calculated based on the *total* physician or QHP time spent on the date of the encounter. Total time includes time spent on both face-to-face and non-face-to-face services.

Additional details of the changes in the calculation of time are provided in Chapter 3.

Revisions to MDM Elements and Definitions

The MDM elements have undergone significant revision for 2021, and extensive clarification is provided in the guidelines to define each element. Clarifications and/or new concepts include:

- Removal of ambiguous terms (eg, *mild*) and definition of previously ambiguous concepts (eg, *acute or chronic illness with systemic symptoms*).
- Definition of important new terms (eg, *independent historian*).
- Redefinition of the data element to expand beyond a simple number of tasks performed and to distinctly acknowledge independent interpretation of tests, as well as discussion of management or test interpretation with an external physician or other QHP.

Additional details of the changes to the MDM elements and definitions are provided in Chapter 2.

Guidelines for New and Revised E/M Codes and Existing E/M Codes

The changes described thus far pertain only to E/M office or other outpatient visit codes, not to other E/M service codes. When referring to the E/M guidelines in 2021, it is important to select the appropriate group of guidelines for each code. This distinction will be particularly important for E/M codes that include MDM in their selection, as the guidelines include two sets of MDM criteria. Table 2 provides a list of E/M categories that use MDM, identifying the codes that have been revised for 2021. A complete list of the E/M codes and guidelines is available in Section 5.

Table 3 provides a summary of the differences in the component(s) for code selection and in the guidelines for E/M office or other outpatient services and other E/M services. Users should ensure that they follow the appropriate set of criteria and guidelines when evaluating services provided in a given code category.

Just as the E/M guidelines differ for office or other outpatient visit codes compared to all other E/M codes, the structure of the E/M guidelines themselves has been revised to accommodate the changes. The structure now contains a segment that is common to all E/M categories and segments that are category specific.

TABLE 2 E/M Services and Medical Decision Making

Category	Subcategory	CPT Codes	Use Existing MDM Criteria	Use Revised 2021 MDM Criteria
Office or Other Outpatient Services				
	New Patient	99202-99205		•
	Established Patient	99211-99215		•
Hospital Observation Services				
	Observation Care Discharge Services	99217		
	Initial Observation Care	99218-99220	•	
	Subsequent Observation Care	99224-99226	•	
Hospital Inpatient Services				
	Initial Hospital Care	99221-99223	•	
	Subsequent Hospital Care	99231-99233	•	
	Observation or Inpatient Care Services (Including Admission and Discharge Services)	99234- 99236	•	
	Hospital Discharge Services	99238-99239		
Consultations				
	Office or Other Outpatient	99241-99245	•	
	Inpatient	99251-99255	•	
Emergency Department Services				
	New or Established Patient	99281-99285	•	
	Other Emergency Services	99288		
Critical Care Services				
	Time-based Critical Care	99291, 99292		
Nursing Facility Services				
	Initial Nursing Facility Care	99304-99306	•	
	Subsequent Nursing Facility Care	99307-99310	•	
	Nursing Facility Discharge Services	99315-99316		
	Other Nursing Facility Services	99318	•	
Domiciliary, Rest Home (eg, Boarding Home), or Custodial Care Services				
	New Patient	99324-99328	•	
	Established Patient	99334-99337	•	
Domiciliary, Rest Home (eg, Assisted Living Facility), or Home Care Plan Oversight Services		99339-99340		
Home Services				
	New Patient	99341-99345	•	
	Established Patient	99347-99350	•	

TABLE 3 Summary of Guideline Differences

►Summary of Guideline Differences◄

►Component(s) for Code Selection	Office or Other Outpatient Services	Other E/M Services (Hospital Observation, Hospital Inpatient, Consultations, Emergency Department, Nursing Facility, Domiciliary, Rest Home, or Custodial Care, Home)
History and Examination	• As medically appropriate. Not used in code selection	• Use key components (history, examination, MDM)
Medical Decision Making (MDM)	• May use MDM or total time on the date of the encounter	• Use key components (history, examination, MDM)
Time	• May use MDM or total time on the date of the encounter	• May use face-to-face time or time at the bedside and on the patient's floor or unit when counseling and/or coordination of care dominates the service. *Time is* ***not*** *a descriptive component for the emergency department levels of E/M services.*
MDM Elements	• Number and complexity of problems addressed at the encounter • Amount and/or complexity of data to be reviewed and analyzed • Risk of complications and/or morbidity or mortality of patient management	• Number of diagnoses or management options • Amount and/or complexity of data to be reviewed • Risk of complications and/or morbidity or mortality◄

Figure 3 shows the current (2020) structure of the E/M guidelines. Figure 4 shows an overview of how various sections of the E/M guidelines have been reorganized and revised for 2021. Figures 3 and 4 provide a quick at-a-glance view of the E/M guidelines' structure, which can be used as a navigation guide, as needed.

For additional navigational assistance, Appendix A, Tabular Review of Changes, contains the detailed changes, additions, and deletions made in the E/M guidelines.

FIGURE 3 E/M Guideline Structure for 2020

Classification of E/M Services
Definitions of Commonly Used Terms
New and Established Patient
Chief Complaint
Concurrent Care and Transfer of Care
Counseling
Family History
History of Present Illness
Levels of E/M Services
Nature of Presenting Problem
Past History
Social History
System Review (Review of Systems)
Time
Unlisted Service
Special Report
Clinical Examples
Instructions for Selecting a Level of E/M Service
Review the Reporting Instructions for the Selected Category or Subcategory
Review E/M Service Descriptors and Examples
Determine the Extent of History Obtained
Determine the Extent of Examination Performed
Determine the Complexity of Medical Decision Making
Select the Appropriate Level of E/M Services

FIGURE 4 Revised E/M Guideline Structure for 2021

E/M Guidelines Overview
Classification of E/M Services
Definitions of Commonly Used Terms
Guidelines Common to All E/M Services
Levels of E/M Services
New and Established Patient
Time
Concurrent Care and Transfer of Care
Counseling
Services Reported Separately
Guidelines for Hospital Observation, Hospital Inpatient, Consultations, Emergency Department, Nursing Facility, Domiciliary, Rest Home, or Custodial Care, and Home E/M Services
Levels of E/M Services
Chief Complaint
History of Present Illness
Levels of E/M Services
Nature of Presenting Problem
Past History
Family History
Social History
System Review (Review of Systems)
Instructions for Selecting a Level of E/M Service for Hospital Observation, Hospital Inpatient, Consultations, Emergency Department, Nursing Facility, Domiciliary, Rest Home, or Custodial Care, and Home E/M Service
Review the Level of E/M Service Descriptors and Examples in the Selected Category or Subcategory
Determine the Extent of History Obtained
Determine the Extent of Examination Performed
Determine the Complexity of Medical Decision Making
Select the Appropriate Level of E/M Services Based on the Following
Guidelines for Office or Other Outpatient E/M Services
History and/or Examination
Number and Complexity of Problems Addressed at the Encounter
Instructions for Selecting a Level of Office or Other Outpatient E/M Services
Medical Decision Making
Time
Unlisted Service
Special Report
Clinical Examples

Evaluate Your Understanding

The following questions and case studies are critical checkpoints that are meant to let you apply your critical thinking and evaluate your understanding of the content covered in the chapter. The answers for the end-of-chapter exercises are available at amaproductupdates.org.

A Multiple Choice Questions

Select the correct or most appropriate answer(s) to the following questions.

1. Which of the following section(s) has been significantly changed in the CPT E/M 2021 section?
   a. Consultations
   b. Hospital Observation Services
   c. Office or Other Outpatient Services
   d. Emergency Department Services

2. What are some of the principal reasons considered in changing the office or other outpatient visit E/M codes for 2021?
   a. Patients over Paperwork
   b. Administrative simplification
   c. A and B
   d. ICD-9-CM was changed to ICD-10-CM

3. What was the catalyst for the 2021 E/M office or outpatient services changes?
   a. Medicare 2019 Physician Fee Schedule
   b. HIPAA
   c. PAMA
   d. AMA

4. Which of the following are some of the key changes in the office or other outpatient visit E/M codes?
   a. Elimination of history and/or physical examination as a component for code selection
   b. Changes in the definitions of MDM and time when used to report office or other outpatient services codes
   c. Deletion of code 99202
   d. A and B

5. Which prolonged services code has been added for 2021?
   a. 99416
   b. 99358
   c. 99355
   d. None of the above

B True/False Questions

Answer true (T) or false (F) to the following statements.

1. _____ Codes 99201 and 99211 have been deleted in 2021.

2. _____ The prolonged service code 99417 may be reported in conjunction with codes 99202-99215.

3. _____ MDM or time may be used to select the level of office or other outpatient visit E/M service.

4. _____ In 2021, time has been defined as total face-to-face time by the physician or other QHP.

5. _____ The new prolonged service code (99417) may be reported only on the date of the encounter.

6. _____ Code 99417 may be reported when both MDM and time are the basis for code selection.

7. _____ The letter sent to CMS in response to the Proposed Rule was signed by 500 organizations.

8. _____ CMS finalized the decision to accept and implement the revisions to the CPT office or other outpatient visit E/M codes on October 1, 2019.

C Fill in the Blank

Fill in the blank in the following statements with the most correct response.

1. During an office visit in 2021, ____________ and ____________ are performed as clinically appropriate, but are not part of the code selection components.
2. CPT code 99201 has been deleted in 2021 because both codes 99201 and 99202 have straightforward MDM and differ only in the ____________ and ____________ elements.
3. Time component reported in 2021 includes ____________ time on the date of the encounter.
4. Revisions to the MDM elements and definitions in 2021 include the new term ____________ and its definition.
5. The revisions to the E/M guidelines in 2021 apply to codes ____________ through ____________ only.
6. Changes to E/M codes for 2021 have been implemented primarily to decrease ____________ burden.
7. The date (month and year) when the road to the 2021 E/M changes began in earnest was ____________.
8. The E/M code–revision efforts of the Relative Value Scale (RVS) Update Committee (RUC) E/M Workgroup were guided by four principles of ____________.

D Internet-based Exercises

1. For more information about Medicare Physician Fee Schedule, visit https://www.cms.gov/Medicare/Medicare-Fee-for-Service-Payment/PhysicianFeeSched.
2. To learn more about RUC, visit https://www.ama-assn.org/about/rvs-update-committee-ruc.
3. Read an article relating to how the 2021 E/M guidelines could ease physicians' documentation burdens at https://www.ama-assn.org/practice-management/cpt/how-2021-em-guidelines-could-ease-physicians-documentation-burdens.
4. To learn more about published proposed rules, visit the *Federal Register* website at https://www.federalregister.gov/.
5. For information about the CPT Editorial Panel, visit https://www.ama-assn.org/about/cpt-editorial-panel.

SECTION 2

E/M 2021: MDM and Code-Level Selection Changes

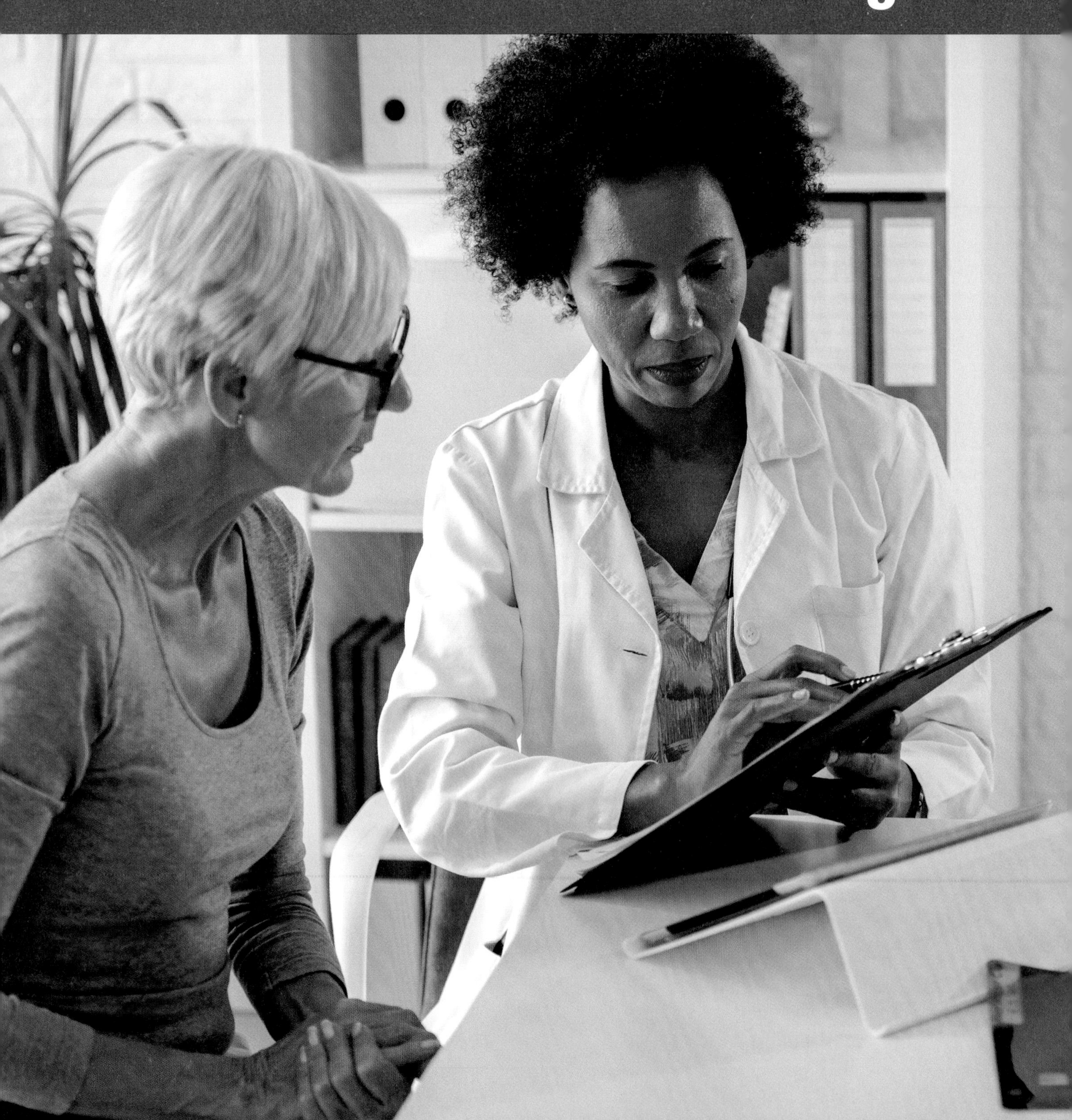

This section offers an in-depth look at the changes implemented for medical decision making (MDM), an important component of the evaluation and management (E/M) guidelines and code descriptors. It guides the reader through the various levels of complexity of MDM, the elements that define each level, and the types of problems that are often involved at each level.

The objectives of this section are as follows:

- Understand every related code revision, with associated criteria and descriptions
- Learn how factors such as the number of problems addressed and the complexity of these problems determine the MDM complexity level
- Master the data element with helpful matrices
- Understand and evaluate the risk element

CHAPTER 2

Medical Decision Making

Physician or other qualified health care professional (QHP)
An individual who is qualified by education, training, licensure/regulation (when applicable), and facility privileging (when applicable) who performs a professional service within the individual's scope of practice and independently reports that professional service.

Medical decision making (MDM)
The complexity of establishing a diagnosis and/or selecting a management option.

Overview

One of the most significant areas of change in the Current Procedural Terminology (CPT®) 2021 code set is the ability of physicians and/or other qualified health care professionals (QHPs) to use either time or medical decision making (MDM) as a primary criterion for code selection.

Prior to 2021, MDM was one of the required key components, along with history and physical examination, used to select the appropriate E/M code level for office or other outpatient visits.

Before 2021, MDM for all E/M codes referred to the complexity of establishing a diagnosis and/or selecting a management option, as measured by:

- The number of diagnoses or management options
- The amount and/or complexity of data to be reviewed
- The risk of complications and/or morbidity or mortality

Within each of these elements, four types of MDM were recognized: straightforward, low complexity, moderate complexity, and high complexity. To qualify for a given level of MDM, two of the three elements in the column headers of Table 1 had to be met or exceeded.

The MDM complexity levels prior to January 1, 2021, are listed in Table 1. This table will continue to define MDM for all but the E/M office or other outpatient codes in 2021.

Specific criteria used to determine a given complexity level for each element have been clarified in the 2021 revisions. Previously, the lack of specific criteria within the CPT code set has contributed to variations in interpretation of the complexity levels across contractors and payers.

TABLE 1 Complexity of Medical Decision Making (Before 2021)

Number of Diagnoses or Management Options	Amount and/or Complexity of Data to be Reviewed	Risk of Complications and/or Morbidity or Mortality	Type of Decision Making
minimal	minimal or none	minimal	**straightforward**
limited	limited	low	**low complexity**
multiple	moderate	moderate	**moderate complexity**
extensive	extensive	high	**high complexity**

Note: Before January 1, 2021, these levels were effective for all E/M codes. Starting January 1, 2021, these levels will be effective for all but E/M office or other outpatient codes.

Summary of Revisions

For E/M office or other outpatient visit codes for 2021, the four types of MDM (straightforward, low complexity, moderate complexity, and high complexity) are unchanged, and MDM is still not necessary for code 99211. Code 99201 has been deleted because the elimination of required history and physical examination elements resulted in a lack of distinction between codes 99201 and 99202.

Additional detail has been added within the revised MDM guidelines to reduce the variation encountered in interpretation of existing MDM levels across contractors and payers. Existing Centers for Medicare & Medicaid Services (CMS) and contractor tables and audit tools have been reviewed to minimize disruption in coding patterns.

One of the most visible changes for 2021 is the new, expanded MDM table for E/M office or other outpatient visit codes. The table incorporates several new features to facilitate proper code selection, including:

- Revised element headers, reflecting refinements made in each category (see Table 2)
- CPT codes incorporated into the table, with codes 99202-99205 and 99211-99215 placed at their appropriate MDM level
- Criteria added at each element level, providing increased clarity to facilitate code selection (see Table 3)

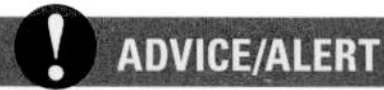

Be sure to consult the official E/M guidelines in the CPT 2021 code set for a full list of element terms and definitions.

Each element included in MDM has been enhanced for 2021. Users should thoroughly familiarize themselves with the changes, including the new definitions outlined in the following sections.

TABLE 2 Changes to Medical Decision Making

MDM Before 2021	MDM Effective January 1, 2021
Number of diagnoses or management options	Number and **complexity of problems addressed at the encounter**
Amount and/or complexity of data to be reviewed	Amount and/or complexity of data to be reviewed **and analyzed**
Risk of complications and/or morbidity or mortality	Risk of complications and/or morbidity or mortality **of patient management**

Medical Decision Making

TABLE 3 Levels of Medical Decision Making (MDM)

▶Table 2: Levels of Medical Decision Making (MDM)◀

▶Code	Level of MDM (Based on 2 out of 3 Elements of MDM)	Elements of Medical Decision Making: Number and Complexity of Problems Addressed at the Encounter	Amount and/or Complexity of Data to be Reviewed and Analyzed **Each unique test, order, or document contributes to the combination of 2 or combination of 3 in Category 1 below.*	Risk of Complications and/or Morbidity or Mortality of Patient Management
99211	N/A	N/A	N/A	N/A
99202 99212	**Straightforward**	**Minimal** • **1** self-limited or minor problem	**Minimal or none**	**Minimal risk of morbidity from additional diagnostic testing or treatment**
99203 99213	**Low**	**Low** • **2** or more self-limited or minor problems; **or** • **1** stable, chronic illness; **or** • **1** acute, uncomplicated illness or injury	**Limited** *(Must meet the requirements of at least 1 of the 2 categories)* **Category 1: Tests and documents** • **Any combination of 2 from the following:** ■ Review of prior external note(s) from each unique source*; ■ Review of the result(s) of each unique test*; ■ Ordering of each unique test* **or** **Category 2: Assessment requiring an independent historian(s)** *(For the categories of independent interpretation of tests and discussion of management or test interpretation, see moderate or high)*	**Low risk of morbidity from additional diagnostic testing or treatment**
99204 99214	**Moderate**	**Moderate** • **1** or more chronic illnesses with exacerbation, progression, or side effects of treatment; **or** • **2** or more stable, chronic illnesses; **or** • **1** undiagnosed new problem with uncertain prognosis; **or** • **1** acute illness with systemic symptoms; **or** • **1** acute, complicated injury	**Moderate** *(Must meet the requirements of at least 1 out of 3 categories)* **Category 1: Tests, documents, or independent historian(s)** • **Any combination of 3 from the following:** ■ Review of prior external note(s) from each unique source*; ■ Review of the result(s) of each unique test*; ■ Ordering of each unique test*; ■ Assessment requiring an independent historian(s) **or** **Category 2: Independent interpretation of tests** • Independent interpretation of a test performed by another physician/other qualified health care professional (not separately reported); **or** **Category 3: Discussion of management or test interpretation** • Discussion of management or test interpretation with external physician/other qualified health care professional/appropriate source (not separately reported)	**Moderate risk of morbidity from additional diagnostic testing or treatment** *Examples only:* • Prescription drug management • Decision regarding minor surgery with identified patient or procedure risk factors • Decision regarding elective major surgery without identified patient or procedure risk factors • Diagnosis or treatment significantly limited by social determinants of health

Code	Level of MDM (Based on 2 out of 3 Elements of MDM)	Elements of Medical Decision Making		
		Number and Complexity of Problems Addressed at the Encounter	**Amount and/or Complexity of Data to be Reviewed and Analyzed** ***Each unique test, order, or document contributes to the combination of 2 or combination of 3 in Category 1 below.**	**Risk of Complications and/or Morbidity or Mortality of Patient Management**
99205 **99215**	**High**	**High** • **1** or more chronic illnesses with severe exacerbation, progression, or side effects of treatment; **or** • **1** acute or chronic illness or injury that poses a threat to life or bodily function	**Extensive** *(Must meet the requirements of at least 2 out of 3 categories)* **Category 1: Tests, documents, or independent historian(s)** • **Any combination of 3 from the following:** ▪ Review of prior external note(s) from each unique source*; ▪ Review of the result(s) of each unique test*; ▪ Ordering of each unique test*; ▪ Assessment requiring an independent historian(s) **or** **Category 2: Independent interpretation of tests** • Independent interpretation of a test performed by another physician/other qualified health care professional (not separately reported); **or** **Category 3: Discussion of management or test interpretation** • Discussion of management or test interpretation with external physician/other qualified health care professional/appropriate source (not separately reported)	**High risk of morbidity from additional diagnostic testing or treatment** *Examples only:* • Drug therapy requiring intensive monitoring for toxicity • Decision regarding elective major surgery with identified patient or procedure risk factors • Decision regarding emergency major surgery • Decision regarding hospitalization • Decision not to resuscitate or to de-escalate care because of poor prognosis◀

MDM Element: Number and Complexity of Problems Addressed at the Encounter

This element was previously titled "Number of Diagnoses or Management Options." Changes made to this element focused on providing clear definitions for each level of MDM outlined in Table 4. Examples previously included in the CMS Table of Risk were reviewed for applicability to the office or outpatient setting; some have been moved to the guidelines to make the MDM table less complex. The resulting structure clearly presents the criteria that are required for each MDM level if this element is used (along with at least one other element) to select an E/M code. To guide selection and reflect the different types of patients seen, each MDM level has examples of types of patients or conditions that are addressed.

ADVICE/ALERT NOTE

In the element "Amount and/or Complexity of Data to be Reviewed and Analyzed," each unique test, order, or document contributes to the combination of two or three components in the Category 1 listings. *A chemistry or other test panel is counted as one unique test.*

TABLE 4 Number and Complexity of Problems Addressed at the Encounter: Criteria and Options

CPT Code	Level of MDM	Number and Complexity of Problems Addressed at the Encounter: Criteria
99211	N/A	N/A
99202 99212	Straightforward	Minimal • 1 self-limited or minor problem
99203 99213	Low	Low • 2 or more self-limited or minor problems *or* • 1 stable chronic illness *or* • 1 acute, uncomplicated illness or injury
99204 99214	Moderate	Moderate • 1 or more chronic illnesses with exacerbation, progression, or side effects of treatment *or* • 2 or more stable chronic illnesses *or* • undiagnosed new problem with uncertain prognosis *or* • 1 acute illness with systemic symptoms *or* • 1 acute complicated injury
99205 99215	High	High • 1 or more chronic illnesses with severe exacerbation, progression, or side effects of treatment *or* • 1 acute or chronic illness or injury that poses a threat to life or bodily function

ADVICE/ALERT NOTE

Understanding Terms: *Problem* vs *Problem Addressed*

- ***Problem:*** In the 2021 E/M guidelines, a *problem* is defined as a disease, condition, illness, injury, symptom, sign, finding, complaint, or other matter noted at the encounter, with or without a diagnosis being established at the time of the encounter.
- ***Problem Addressed or Managed:*** A problem is considered to be *addressed or managed* when it is evaluated or treated at the encounter by the physician or other QHP reporting the service. This includes consideration of further testing or treatment that may not be elected by virtue of risk-benefit analysis or patient, parent, guardian, or surrogate choice.

Key Definitions and Examples

The 2021 E/M guidelines provide additional clarity on definitions of all the criteria. Key changes include clarification of the term *problem* and when a problem is considered to be *addressed*. The distinction between these two terms is central to identifying activities that can be counted toward meeting the criteria for this element.

- In the 2021 E/M guidelines, a *problem* is defined as a disease, condition, illness, injury, symptom, sign, finding, complaint, or other matter noted at the encounter, with or without a diagnosis being established at the time of the encounter.
- A problem is considered to be *addressed or managed* when it is evaluated or treated at the encounter by the physician or other QHP reporting the service. This includes consideration of further testing or treatment that may not be elected by virtue of risk-benefit analysis or patient, parent, guardian, or surrogate choice.

Situations that *do not* qualify as being addressed or managed by the physician or other QHP reporting the service include the following:

- Notation in the patient's medical record that another professional is managing the problem without documenting additional assessment or care coordination
- Referral without evaluation (by history, examination, or diagnostic study[ies] or consideration of treatment)
- Other diagnoses or conditions that the patient has but that are not addressed in the encounter

Table 5 provides concrete descriptions and clinical examples of the criteria used in choosing an E/M code associated with a given MDM level.

ADVICE/ALERT NOTE

Comorbidities and/or underlying diseases, in and of themselves, are not considered in selecting a level of E/M service *unless* they are addressed *and* their presence increases the amount and/or complexity of data to be reviewed and analyzed or the risk of complications and/or morbidity or mortality of patient management.

TABLE 5 Problems, Illnesses, and Injuries: Definitions and Examples

MDM Level	Criterion	Description	Example
Straightforward	Self-limited or minor problem	A problem that runs a definite and prescribed course, is transient in nature, and is not likely to permanently alter health status.	
Low	Stable, chronic illness	A problem with an expected duration of at least 1 year or until the death of the patient. • For the purpose of defining chronicity, conditions are treated as chronic whether or not stage or severity changes (eg, uncontrolled diabetes and controlled diabetes are a single chronic condition). • "Stable" for the purposes of categorizing MDM is defined by the specific treatment goals for an individual patient. A patient who is not at their treatment goal is not stable, even if the condition has not changed and there is no short-term threat to life or function. For example, a patient with persistently poorly controlled blood pressure for whom better control is a goal is not stable, even if the pressures are not changing and the patient is asymptomatic, the risk of morbidity **without** treatment is significant.	Well-controlled hypertension, non-insulin-dependent diabetes, cataract, or benign prostatic hyperplasia
	Acute, uncomplicated illness or injury	A recent or new short-term problem with low risk of morbidity for which treatment is considered. There is little to no risk of mortality with treatment, and full recovery without functional impairment is expected. A problem that is normally self-limited or minor but is not resolving consistent with a definite and prescribed course is an acute uncomplicated illness.	Cystitis, allergic rhinitis, simple sprain

(continued)

TABLE 5 Problems, Illnesses, and Injuries: Definitions and Examples, *continued*

MDM Level	Criterion	Description	Example
Moderate	Chronic illness with exacerbation, progression, or side effects of treatment	A chronic illness that is acutely worsening, poorly controlled, or progressing with an intent to control progression and requiring additional supportive care or requiring attention to treatment for side effects but does not require consideration of hospital level of care.	Asthma exacerbation
	Undiagnosed new problem with uncertain prognosis	A problem in the differential diagnosis that represents a condition likely to result in a high risk of morbidity without treatment.	Breast lump
	Acute illness with systemic symptoms	An illness that causes systemic symptoms and has a high risk of morbidity without treatment. For systemic general symptoms such as fever, body aches, or fatigue in a minor illness that may be treated to alleviate symptoms, shorten the course of an illness, or prevent complications, see the definitions for **self-limited or minor problem** or **acute, uncomplicated illness or injury.** Systemic symptoms may not be general but may be single system.	Pyelonephritis, pneumonitis, or colitis
	Acute, complicated injury	An injury which requires treatment that includes evaluation of body systems that are not directly a part of the injured organ, the injury is extensive, or the treatment options are multiple and/or associated with a risk of morbidity.	Head injury with brief loss of consciousness
High	Chronic illness with severe exacerbation, progression, or side effects of treatment	The severe exacerbation or progression of a chronic illness or severe side effects of treatment that have significant risk of morbidity and may require hospital level of care.	Chronic obstructive pulmonary disease exacerbation
	Acute or chronic illness or injury that poses a threat to life or bodily function	An acute illness with systemic symptoms, an acute complicated injury, or a chronic illness or injury with exacerbation and/or progression or side effects of treatment, that poses a threat to life or bodily function in the near term without treatment.	Acute myocardial infarction, pulmonary embolus, severe respiratory distress, progressive severe rheumatoid arthritis, psychiatric illness with potential threat to self or others, peritonitis, acute renal failure, an abrupt change in neurologic status

MDM Element: Amount and/or Complexity of Data to be Reviewed and Analyzed

This element was previously titled "Amount and/or Complexity of Data to be Reviewed." Revisions and enhancements to this element focus on simplifying and standardizing scoring guidelines and increasing emphasis on activities that affect patient care beyond the number of documents or test results reviewed. (See Table 6.) This emphasis is expressed through two key changes:

1. An expanded definition of data in the 2021 guidelines: "Data include medical records, tests, and/or other information that must be obtained, ordered, reviewed, and analyzed for the encounter."
2. The introduction of criteria categories each representing a different type of data and work required by the physician or other QHP, utilized in evaluating the patient.

ADVICE/ALERT NOTE

Under the element "Amount and/or Complexity of Data to be Reviewed and Analyzed," each unique test, order, or document contributes to the combination of two or three components in the Category 1 listings. *A panel is considered one unique test.*

TABLE 6 MDM Element Criteria: Amount and/or Complexity of Data to be Reviewed and Analyzed

Code	MDM Level	Amount and/or Complexity of Data to be Reviewed and Analyzed ** Each unique test, order, or document contributes to the combination of 2 or combination of 3 in Category 1 below.*
99211	N/A	N/A
99202 **99212**	Straightforward	Minimal or none
99203 **99213**	Low	Limited *(Must meet the requirements of at least 1 of the 2 categories)* Category 1: Tests and documents • Any combination of 2 from the following: ▪ Review of prior external note(s) from each unique source*; ▪ Review of the result(s) of each unique test*; ▪ Ordering of each unique test* *or* Category 2: Assessment requiring an independent historian(s) (For the categories of independent interpretation of tests and discussion of management or test interpretation, see moderate or high)

(continued)

TABLE 6 MDM Element Criteria: Amount and/or Complexity of Data to be Reviewed and Analyzed, *continued*

Code	MDM Level	**Amount and/or Complexity of Data to be Reviewed and Analyzed** ** Each unique test, order, or document contributes to the combination of 2 or combination of 3 in Category 1 below.*
99204 **99214**	Moderate	Moderate *(Must meet the requirements of at least 1 out of 3 categories)* Category 1: Tests, documents, or independent historian(s) • Any combination of 3 from the following: ▪ Review of prior external note(s) from each unique source*; ▪ Review of the result(s) of each unique test*; ▪ Ordering of each unique test*; ▪ Assessment requiring an independent historian(s) *or* Category 2: Independent interpretation of tests • Independent interpretation of a test performed by another physician/other qualified health care professional (not separately reported); *or* Category 3: Discussion of management or test interpretation • Discussion of management or test interpretation with external physician/other qualified health care professional/appropriate source (not separately reported)
99205 **99215**	High	Extensive *(Must meet the requirements of at least 2 out of 3 categories)* Category 1: Tests, documents, or independent historian(s) • Any combination of 3 from the following: ▪ Review of prior external note(s) from each unique source*; ▪ Review of the result(s) of each unique test*; ▪ Ordering of each unique test*; ▪ Assessment requiring an independent historian(s) *or* Category 2: Independent interpretation of tests • Independent interpretation of a test performed by another physician/other qualified health care professional (not separately reported); *or* Category 3: Discussion of management or test interpretation • Discussion of management or test interpretation with external physician/other qualified health care professional/appropriate source (not separately reported)

Key Definitions and Reporting Considerations

Revisions in the data element include a number of definitions for key and new terms, as well as considerations for reporting, which should be studied to ensure that the criteria are appropriately applied.

Data Element Category 1: Tests, Documents, or Independent Historians

Category 1 in Table 6 outlines criteria related to tests, documents, and orders for all MDM levels. For moderate and high levels of MDM, an option for assessment of a problem, illness, or injury requiring the participation of an independent historian is also included. Taken together, these activities emphasize clinical work beyond just counting the number of documents reviewed. Key terms from this category have been clarified in the 2021 guidelines and are shown in Table 7.

TABLE 7 Tests, Documents, and Independent Historians: Terms and Definitions

Term	Definition
Test	Tests are services that result in imaging, laboratory, psychometric, or physiologic data. The differentiation between single and multiple unique tests is defined in accordance with the CPT code set. When a CPT code representing a clinical laboratory panel is reported (eg, CPT code 80047, *Basic metabolic panel (Calcium, ionized))*, it is considered a single test.
External	External records, communications, and/or test results are from an external physician, other qualified health care professional, facility, or health care organization.
Independent historian(s)	An independent historian is an individual (eg, parent, guardian, surrogate, spouse, witness) who provides a history in addition to the history provided by the patient who is unable to provide a complete or reliable history (eg, due to developmental stage, dementia, or psychosis) or because a confirmatory history is judged to be necessary. Key to this definition is that the independent historian should provide additional information, and not merely restate information already provided by the patient.

New key reporting considerations should be noted for tests and independent historians. The 2021 guidelines state: "Ordering a test is included in the category of test result(s) and the review of the test result is part of the encounter and not a subsequent encounter." For independent historians, the 2021 guidelines state: "In the case where there may be conflict or poor communication between multiple historians and more than one historian is needed, the independent historian requirement is met."

CODING TIP When a test is ordered and results are reviewed as part of an encounter, it is counted as only one completed item in the data element.

Data Element Category 2: Independent Interpretation of Tests

This category addresses the work performed in the E/M physician's or other QHP's independent interpretation of a test that has not been separately reported by the physician or other QHP providing the E/M service. Key reporting considerations include the following:

1. The test should be one for which there is a CPT code and an interpretation or report is customary.
2. A form of independent interpretation should be documented by the physician or other QHP reporting the E/M service, but does not have to conform to the usual standards of a complete report for the test.
3. This criterion is not to be applied when the physician or other QHP is reporting the service or has previously reported the service for the patient.

This criterion would be met in a situation such as the following:

- Dr A conducts an initial office visit for a 12-week-old with bilateral hip dislocations and bilateral club feet. During the visit, Dr A reviews and documents an independent interpretation of X rays that were taken at another facility before the patient came under Dr A's care. In this case, the criterion of independent interpretation of tests has been met.

This criterion would not be met in a situation such as the following:

- Dr S conducts an office visit for the biannual follow-up of an established patient with migraine variant having infrequent, intermittent, moderate to severe headaches with nausea and vomiting, which are sometimes effectively managed with the use of ergotamine tartrate and an antiemetic but occasionally require visits to an emergency department. During the visit, Dr S reviews a radiologist's interpretation of a CT scan taken when the patient suffered a severe migraine on a recent out-of-town vacation, but Dr S does not prepare an independent interpretation of the results. In this case, the criterion of independent interpretation of tests has not been met.

Data Element Category 3: Discussion of Management or Test Interpretation

This category recognizes the work performed by the physician or other QHP in discussion of management or test interpretation with an external physician or other QHP or appropriate source. These two groups are more clearly defined in the guidelines and in Table 8.

TABLE 8 Discussion of Management or Test Interpretation: Definitions

Term	Definition
External physician or other QHP	An external physician or other QHP is one who is not in the same group practice or is of a different specialty or subspecialty. This includes licensed professionals who are practicing independently. The individual may also be a facility or organizational provider such as from a hospital, nursing facility, or home health care agency.
Appropriate source	In this element, an appropriate source includes professionals who are not health care professionals but may be involved in the evaluation and management of the patient's problem (eg, lawyer, parole officer, case manager, teacher). It does not include discussion with family or informal caregivers.

A key reporting consideration is that, when the physician or other QHP is reporting a separate service for discussion of management with an external physician or QHP, the time and/or work involved in reporting that separate service is not counted toward MDM in the selection of a level of office or other outpatient service. The following examples illustrate this distinction:

- Dr J, a family practice physician, conducts an office visit for a 68-year-old female established patient for routine review and follow-up of non-insulin-dependent diabetes, obesity, hypercholesterolemia, hypertension, and congestive heart failure. The patient complains of vision difficulties and admits dietary noncompliance. Her A1c value is > 9. During the visit, Dr J confers briefly with Dr A, an endocrinologist in the same group practice, regarding the best next step in pharmacotherapy given the patient's multiple comorbidities. Results of the discussion factor into Dr J's counseling of the patient on diet and adjustment of the patient's medications. This discussion of management is counted toward MDM when Dr J is selecting a level of office or other outpatient service.
- Dr W, also a family practice physician, sees a patient similar to Dr J's patient, but Dr W reports code 99452 for 16-30 minutes in a service day preparing to communicate with a consultant, Dr I, an independently practicing endocrinologist two states away. Dr W could not use this time or work toward establishing a level of MDM for an E/M code reported on the same day.

An example of communication with an appropriate source would be the following:

- Dr D, a family practice physician, communicates with the teacher of a patient who is being treated for attention deficit hyperactivity disorder (ADHD) and a learning disability. The patient's medications were recently adjusted. The teacher reports that the student's work has improved and the student is making progress toward reaching their grade level.

Accurate Criteria Evaluation: Data Element Decision Matrices

Determining the proper level of complexity in the data element requires a series of selections at each category level. The decision trees in Figures 1, 2, and 3 have been created to assist the user in evaluating the requirements and determining the level of complexity that has been met in this element.

The first tree (Figure 1) is for limited level of complexity. The tree presents a number of paths to meet the criteria for limited level of complexity. Within this framework, it is possible to fulfill the requirements for limited level of complexity solely by meeting the independent historian criterion.

The second tree (Figure 2) is for moderate level of complexity, with three criteria categories. For the moderate level of complexity in this element, at least one of the three group criteria needs to be met.

The third tree (Figure 3) is for high level of complexity, with three criteria categories. For the high level of complexity in this element, criteria in two of the three categories need to be met.

FIGURE 1 Decision Tree for Limited Level MDM

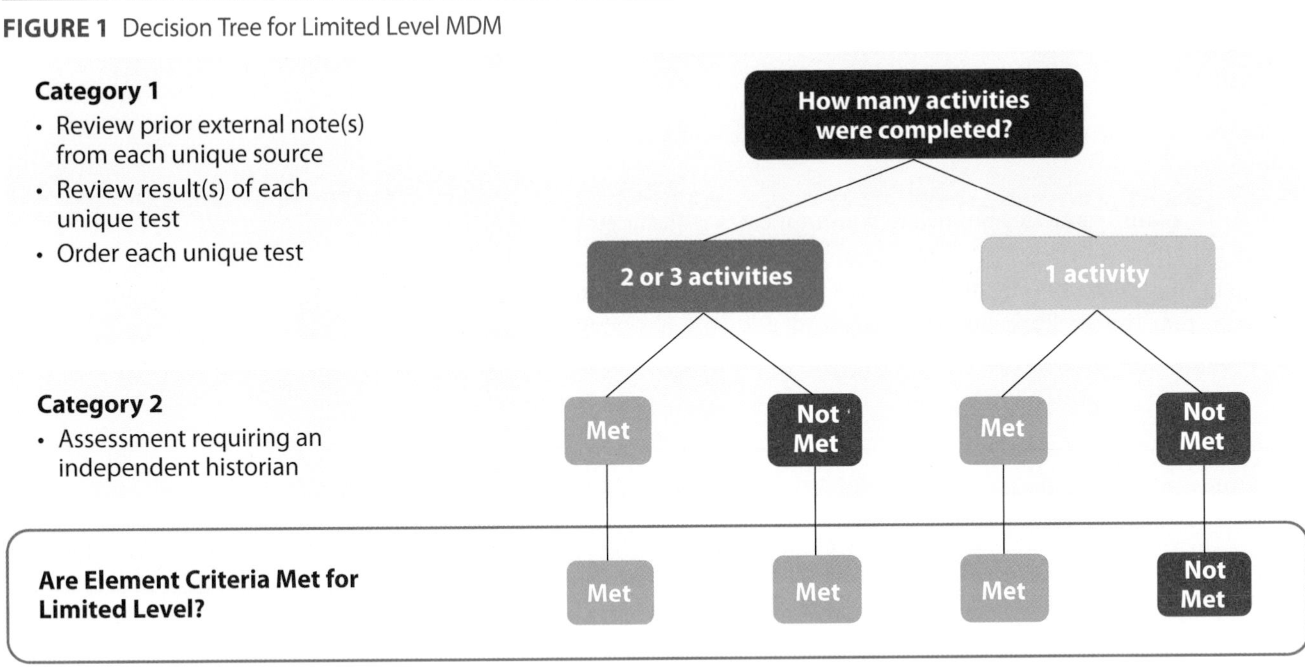

FIGURE 2 Decision Tree for Moderate Level MDM

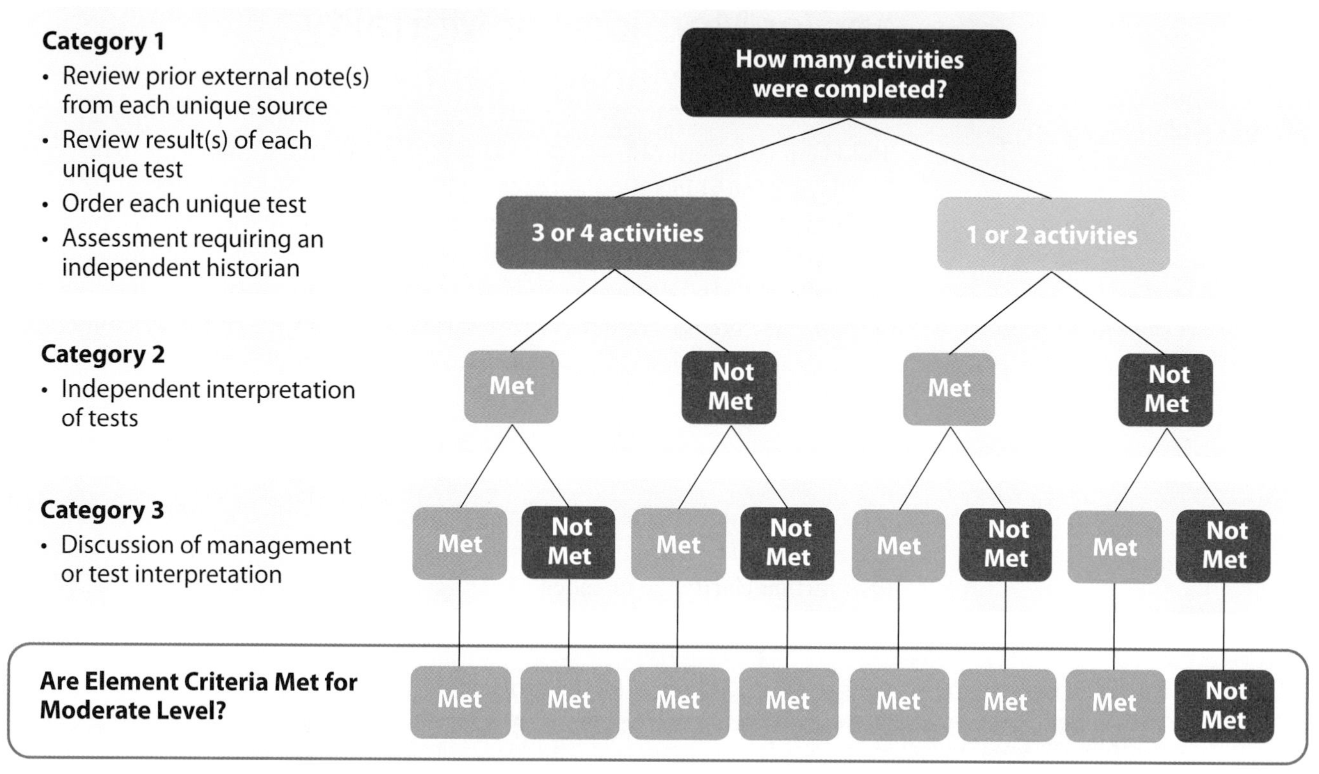

FIGURE 3 Decision Tree for High Level MDM

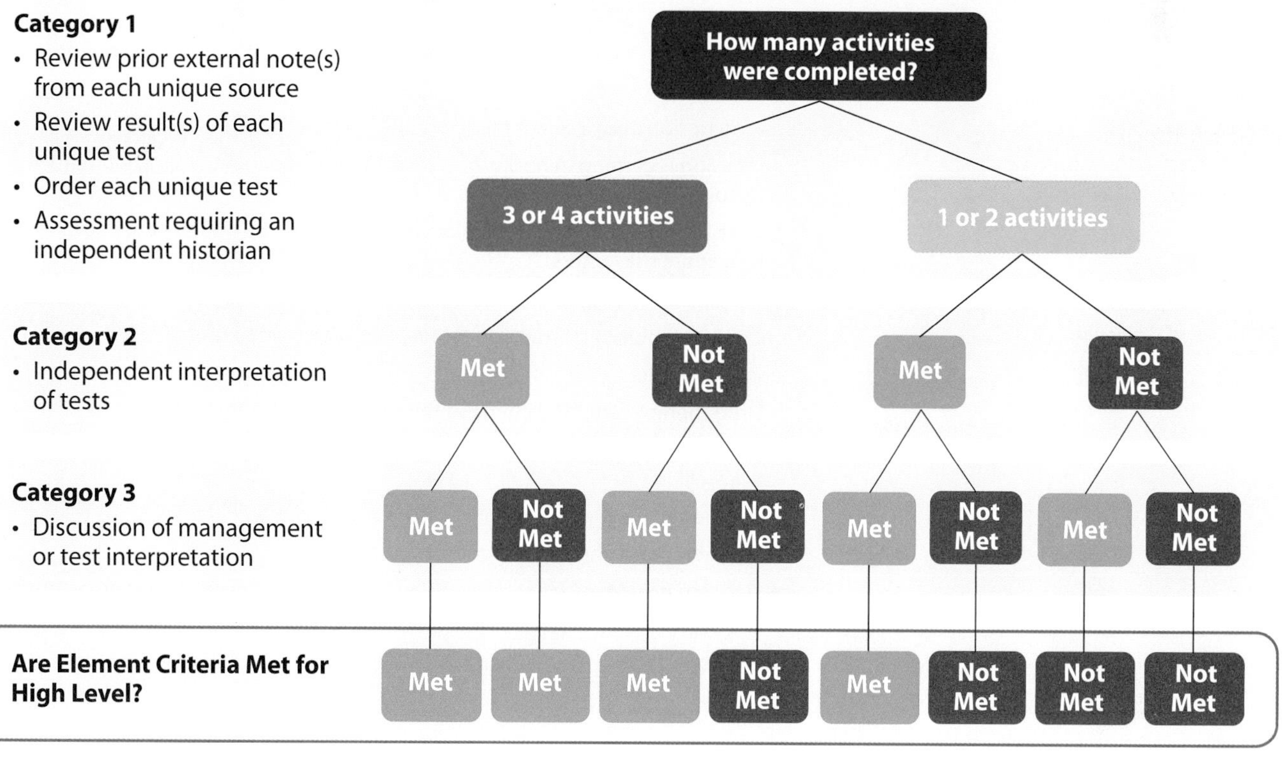

MDM Element: Risk of Complications and/or Morbidity or Mortality of Patient Management

This element was previously titled "Risk of Complications and/or Morbidity or Mortality." The guideline changes for 2021 have increased the emphasis on work performed by the physician or other QHP in addressing patient management decisions made at the visit, associated with the patient's problem(s), diagnostic procedure(s), and treatment(s). Note that this element encompasses the work of both the management options selected and those that were considered but not selected after shared MDM with the patient and/or family.

Changes to Risk Element

Structural changes made to this element focus on providing a more streamlined presentation of terms, with retention of some examples within the table (see Table 9) to further clarify the intended use at the moderate and high levels of MDM.

TABLE 9 Risk of Complications and/or Morbidity or Mortality of Patient Management

CPT Code	Overall MDM Level	Criteria
99211	N/A	N/A
99202 **99212**	Straightforward	Minimal risk of morbidity from additional diagnostic testing or treatment
99203 **99213**	Low	Low risk of morbidity from additional diagnostic testing or treatment
99204 **99214**	Moderate	Moderate risk of morbidity from additional diagnostic testing or treatment Some examples: • Prescription drug management • Decision regarding minor surgery with identified patient or procedure risk factors • Decision regarding elective major surgery without identified patient or procedure risk factors • Diagnosis or treatment significantly limited by social determinants of health
99205 **99215**	High	High risk of morbidity from additional diagnostic testing or treatment Some examples: • Drug therapy requiring intensive monitoring for toxicity • Decision regarding elective major surgery with identified patient or procedure risk factors • Decision regarding emergency major surgery • Decision regarding hospitalization • Decision not to resuscitate or to de-escalate care because of poor prognosis

Similar to the guidelines for the number and complexity of problems addressed at the encounter, the 2021 E/M guidelines provide a clear interpretation of the key concept in this element: the concept of risk.

Risk is the probability and/or consequences of an event. The assessment of the level of risk is affected by the nature of the event under consideration. For example, a low probability of death may be high risk, whereas a high chance of a minor, self-limited adverse effect of treatment may be low risk. (This is because, death, while unlikely, is a possible outcome that is extreme.) Definitions of risk are based on the usual behavior and thought processes of a physician or other QHP in the same specialty; therefore, events that are extremely improbable, such as having an allergic reaction to any antibiotic, would not be counted.

For the purposes of MDM, level of risk is based on consequences of the problem(s) addressed at the encounter when appropriately treated. Risk also includes MDM related to the need to initiate or forgo further testing, treatment, and/or hospitalization. **A key reporting consideration, per the guidelines, is that trained clinicians apply common language-usage meanings to terms such as *high, medium, low,* or *minimal* risk and do not require quantification for these definitions**, though quantification may be provided when evidence-based medicine has established probabilities.

> **ADVICE/ALERT NOTE**
>
> The final diagnosis for a condition does not in itself determine the complexity or risk, as extensive evaluation may be required to reach the conclusion that the signs or symptoms do not represent a highly morbid condition. Multiple problems of a lower severity may, in the aggregate, create a higher risk due to interactions.

Key Definitions and Examples

In addition to risk, four terms in this element are clarified in the 2021 E/M guidelines, along with examples of how to interpret each of them and evaluate whether the criterion has been met.

Shared MDM

Shared MDM involves eliciting patient and/or family preferences, providing patient and/or family education, and explaining risks and benefits of management options. An example of shared MDM would be a decision about hospitalization that includes consideration of alternative levels of care. Other examples may include the decision to manage a psychiatric patient with a sufficient degree of support in the outpatient setting, or the decision not to hospitalize a patient with advanced dementia and an acute condition that would generally warrant inpatient care, but for whom the goal is palliative treatment.

Morbidity

Morbidity is defined as a state of illness or functional impairment that is expected to be of substantial duration during which function is limited, quality of life is impaired, or there is organ damage that may not be transient despite treatment.

Social Determinants of Health

The concept of social determinants of health has been newly clarified in the E/M guidelines for 2021, where it appears as an example of a diagnosis or treatment limitation within the moderate morbidity level. It is defined within the guidelines as "economic and social conditions that influence the health of people and communities"; food and housing insecurity are examples.

ADVICE/ALERT NOTE

The set of ICD-10-CM codes that represent social determinants of health are often referred to as the "Z codes." While these diagnosis codes begin with the letter Z, they are only a subset of a broader set of ICD-10-CM diagnosis codes beginning with Z, "Factors influencing health status and contact with health services" (Z00-Z99).

ADVICE/ALERT NOTE

Contact your third-party payer to determine their documentation and diagnosis code requirements, if any, when using social determinants of health as a criterion for MDM-level selection.

When evaluating level of complexity using this criteria, note that the term *social determinants of health* has been used in many health care contexts. As defined by the World Health Organization, social determinants of health are "the conditions in which people are born, grow, work, live, and age, and the wider set of forces and systems shaping the conditions of daily life, including economic policies and systems, development agendas, social norms, social policies and political systems."[1] The International Classification of Diseases, Tenth Revision, Clinical Modification (ICD-10-CM) diagnosis code set includes a series of codes relating to "Persons with potential health hazards related to socioeconomic and psychosocial circumstances" (Z55-Z65).[2] The codes incorporate conditions beyond housing and food insecurity, including education and literacy, occupational exposure to risk factors, economic circumstances, and other social factors. Documentation requirements for social determinants of health may vary greatly across third-party payers; users should contact the specific payer for their reporting requirements and to determine whether the ICD-10-CM diagnosis codes noted above would be required along with the level of complexity selected.

Social determinants of health are relevant in the context of MDM level selection when they must be considered or affect the decisions regarding management. Like medical comorbidities, they are not considered in selecting a level of E/M services *unless* they are addressed *and* their presence increases the amount and/or complexity of data to be reviewed and analyzed or the risk of complications and/or morbidity or mortality of patient management.

Drug Therapy Requiring Intensive Monitoring for Toxicity

Drug therapy requiring intensive monitoring for toxicity is noted as an example of an activity meeting the criteria for a high level of morbidity. A drug that requires intensive monitoring is a therapeutic agent that has the potential to cause serious morbidity or death. Note that the monitoring is performed for assessment of these adverse effects, not primarily for assessment of therapeutic efficacy. The monitoring should be that which is generally accepted practice for the agent but may be patient-specific in some cases.

In addition to the definition, parameters to further clarify the requirements have been incorporated:

- Intensive monitoring may be long-term or short-term. Long-term intensive monitoring is not performed less than quarterly.
- The monitoring may be performed with a laboratory test, a physiologic test, or imaging.

Monitoring by history or examination does *not* qualify. The monitoring affects the level of MDM in an encounter in which it is considered in the management of the patient.

Examples of monitoring that qualify include:

- Monitoring for cytopenia in the use of an antineoplastic agent between dose cycles
- Short-term intensive monitoring of electrolytes and renal function in a patient who is undergoing diuresis

Examples of monitoring that would not qualify, and the reasons for that determination, include:

- Monitoring of glucose levels during insulin therapy. This would not qualify because the primary reason for monitoring is the therapeutic effect (even if hypoglycemia is a concern).
- Annual electrolytes and renal function for a patient on a diuretic. In this case, the annual frequency does not meet the threshold, so the monitoring would not qualify.

References

1. Robeznieks A. Social determinants of health: What they are, what they aren't. https://www.ama-assn.org/delivering-care/patient-support-advocacy/social-determinants-health-what-they-are-what-they-arent. Accessed July 2, 2020.
2. Centers for Disease Control and Prevention. International Classification of Diseases, Tenth Revision, Clinical Modification (ICD-10-CM). https://www.cdc.gov/nchs/icd/icd10cm.htm. Accessed July 2, 2020.

Evaluate Your Understanding

The following questions and case studies are critical checkpoints that are meant to let you apply your critical thinking and evaluate your understanding of the content covered in the chapter. The answers for the end-of-chapter exercises are available at amaproductupdates.org**.**

A Multiple Choice Questions

Select the correct or most appropriate answer(s) to the following questions.

1. Which of the following is the most accurate definition of **problem** according to the CPT E/M guidelines?
   a. A disease, condition, illness, injury, symptom, sign, finding, complaint, or other matter noted at the encounter with or without a diagnosis being established at the encounter.
   b. Medical decision making regarding a disease
   c. Risk of problems assessed and treated
   d. None of the above

2. What term is used in E/M services to refer to the complexity of establishing a diagnosis and/or selecting a management option?
   a. H&E
   b. MDM
   c. Risk management
   d. None of the above

3. What are the four types or levels of complexity in MDM?
   a. Straightforward, low, medium average, and high
   b. Simple, low, average, and medium
   c. Straightforward, low, moderate, and high
   d. None of the above

4. What is the correct term to describe external records, communications, and/or test results from an external physician, other qualified health care professional, facility, or health care organization?
   a. PHI
   b. Medical documentations
   c. External notes
   d. None of the above

5. What is meant by shared MDM?
   a. Asking questions to fulfill documentation and meaningful use requirements
   b. Eliciting patient and/or family preferences, providing patient and/or family education, and explaining risks and benefits of management options
   c. Eliciting risk associated with a patient's conditions
   d. None of the above

6. Who is considered an "appropriate source" according to the E/M guidelines?
   a. Patient and his or her family and relatives
   b. Professionals who are not health care professionals but may be involved in the evaluation and management of the patient's problem (eg, lawyer, parole officer, case manager, teacher)
   c. Only health care providers
   d. None of the above

7. Which of the following is included as an independent historian and may be given medical power of attorney for a patient?
   a. Surrogate
   b. Nanny
   c. Replacement
   d. None of the above

8. Which of the following terms is defined as the probability and/or consequences of an event?
   a. H&P
   b. MDM
   c. Risk
   d. None of the above

9. Which of the following terms is defined as services that result in imaging, laboratory, psychometric, or physiologic data?
   a. MDM level
   b. Tests
   c. Risks
   d. None of the above

10. Which of the following terms is defined as individuals (eg, parent, guardian, surrogate, spouse, witness) who provide a history in addition to the history provided by the patient who is unable to provide a complete or reliable history (eg, due to developmental stage, dementia, or psychosis) or because a confirmatory history is judged to be necessary?
   a. Independent historians
   b. Surrogates
   c. Power of attorney
   d. None of the above

11. What is the definition of morbidity?
   a. A state of having a chronic disease without a cure.
   b. A state of having permanent impairment that affects a person's activities of daily living.
   c. A state of illness or functional impairment that is expected to be of substantial duration during which function is limited, quality of life is impaired, or there is organ damage that may not be transient despite treatment.
   d. None of the above

12. Economic and social conditions that influence the health of people and communities are also known as which of the following terms?
   a. Social and health economic disparity
   b. Social determinants of health
   c. Risks to health and emotional well-being
   d. None of the above

B True/False Questions

Answer true (T) or false (F) to the following statements.

1. ______ The four types of MDM recognized for each element are straightforward, low complexity, moderate complexity, and high complexity.

2. ______ The three key risk element terms are morbidity, social determinants of health, and drug therapy requiring intensive monitoring for toxicity.

3. ______ It is appropriate to use MDM for code 99211.

4. ______ Shared MDM involves eliciting patient and/or family preferences, providing patient and/or family education, and explaining risks and benefits of management options.

5. ______ For the purposes of MDM, the level of risk is based on consequences of the problem(s) addressed at the encounter when appropriately treated.

6. ______ A problem is *addressed or managed* when it is evaluated or treated at the encounter by the physician or other qualified health care professional (QHP) reporting the service.

7. ______ In the assessment of the amount and/or complexity of data to be reviewed, the data include medical records, tests, and/or other information that must be obtained, ordered, reviewed, and analyzed for the patient encounter.

8. ______ Ordering a test is not included in the category of test result(s), and the review of the test result is not part of the encounter and is a subsequent encounter.

9. ______ One consideration for the physician's or other QHP's independent interpretation of a test should be a test for which there is a CPT code and an interpretation or report is customary.

10. ______ In the element "Amount and/or Complexity of Data to be Reviewed and Analyzed," each unique test, order, or document contributes to the combination of one or two components in the high MDM Category 1 listing.

11. _____ In 2021, three required key components (history, physical examination, and MDM) are used to select the appropriate E/M level for office or other outpatient services.

12. _____ A patient with stable, chronic illness with well-controlled hypertension, non-insulin-dependent diabetes, cataract, or benign prostatic hyperplasia would qualify for a low MDM level code selection.

C Fill in the Blank

Fill in the blank in the following statements with the most correct response.

1. Physicians and/or other QHPs may use either medical decision making (MDM) or ____________________ as a primary code-selection criterion.
2. MDM measures the number and ____________________ of problems addressed at the encounter.
3. The four types of MDM recognized for each element are ____________________, low complexity, moderate complexity, and high complexity.
4. In 2021, MDM is still not applicable for code ____________________.
5. Code ____________________ has been deleted because there was no distinction between it and code 99202 with the new MDM definitions.
6. In the "Risk of Complications and/or Morbidity or Mortality of Patient Management" column in Table 3, low MDM demonstrates ____________________ risk of morbidity from additional diagnostic testing or treatment.
7. The criteria for ____________________ complexity include one or more chronic illnesses with exacerbation, progression, or side effects of treatment.
8. A problem is addressed or ____________________ when it is evaluated or treated at the encounter by the physician or other QHP reporting the service.
9. An undiagnosed new problem with uncertain prognosis is a criterion for ____________________ MDM.
10. ____________________ and underlying diseases are not considered in selecting a level of E/M service *unless* they are addressed *and* their presence increases the amount and/or complexity of data to be reviewed and analyzed or the risk of complications and/or morbidity or mortality of patient management.
11. For 2021, ____________________ a test is included in the category of test result(s), and the review of the test result is part of the encounter and not a subsequent encounter.
12. An ____________________ physician or other QHP is one who is not in the same group practice or is in a different specialty or subspecialty.

D Internet-based Exercises 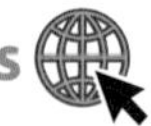

1. For more information about E/M 2021, see https://www.medtronsoftware.com/pdf/newsblasts/061920_E&M_2021_Updates.pdf.
2. For additional information on 2021 E/M changes in MDM, see https://namas.co/2021-em-changes-in-mdm-putting-it-all-together/.
3. For additional information on 2021 changes in risk in MDM, see https://www.doctors-management.com/2021-em-changes-risk-in-the-mdm/.
4. For information on the difference between morbidity and mortality, visit https://www.verywellhealth.com/what-is-morbidity-2223380.
5. For CMS' E/M Services Guide, visit https://www.cms.gov/Outreach-and-Education/Medicare-Learning-Network-MLN/MLNProducts/Downloads/eval-mgmt-serv-guide-ICN006764.pdf.

E Short Answer Questions

Answer the following questions with the most correct response.

1. Does MDM apply to code 99211?
2. In 2021, what elements will be used to select the appropriate E/M office or other outpatient code level?
3. In CPT E/M guidelines, when is a problem considered to be addressed?
4. In CPT E/M guidelines, when comorbidities or underlying diseases exist but are not relevant to the condition being treated, are they still considered when the appropriate E/M code is selected?
5. In CPT E/M guidelines, what are the four types of MDM recognized for each element?
6. Are notes in the medical record from a physician or QHP in another specialty of the same facility considered "external notes"?
7. Does the family always need to participate when patient management options are discussed in order for "shared MDM" to be considered a reportable MDM element?
8. The guidelines for independent interpretation of tests state: "This does not apply when the physician or other qualified health care professional is reporting the service or has previously reported the service for the patient." If I did an X ray 2 months ago in my office and previously reported that service, and now the patient returns with a recent X ray taken in a different facility, does this criterion apply?
9. In the criteria for the data element, "appropriate source" does not include discussion with family or informal caregivers. If an individual has medical power of attorney but is not related to the patient, is this individual considered an "appropriate source"? If no, why not?
10. In the criteria for the data element, is the independent historian requirement met if the historian only translates what the patient has already said?
11. In the criteria for the data element, for "ordering of each unique test," if I order a lab panel, can I count each test in the panel individually in meeting the criteria?
12. With the new MDM guidelines, is there a detailed table to assist in counting the applicable risk factors?

F Case Studies

Although each of the following scenarios may involve service(s) or procedure(s) besides E/M, code only the E/M services. Use the *CPT 2021* codebook to determine the correct code(s) to report the E/M service(s) associated with each of the following procedure(s) or service(s).

Case Study 1

A 64-year-old female patient presents to the office complaining of pain and what she describes as a tingling/burning sensation in her extremities that has been occurring for the past several weeks. She is well known and was otherwise stable, being managed for diabetes mellitus type 2 and hypertension. The physician performs a relevant physical examination and orders a thyroid-stimulating hormone (TSH) test, vitamin B12 test, basic metabolic panel, and A1c test because idiopathic or diabetic peripheral neuropathy leads the differential diagnosis. It is determined that the patient should be evaluated for peripheral neuropathy by a specialist in neurology, and the physician refers the patient for a neurological evaluation while continuing to manage her ongoing, chronic conditions. Which MDM level(s) and E/M code(s) should be reported for this case study?

Case Study 2

A 77-year-old male established patient with severe chronic obstructive pulmonary disease (COPD) who had been using a short-acting bronchodilator inhaler to control his symptoms in addition to his control inhalers came to see his primary care physician emergently because his coughing, wheezing, and shortness of breath had increased more than usual. The physician accessed and reviewed his medical record, including the patient's comorbidities of coronary artery disease and recent weight loss, performed an appropriate physical examination and pulse oximetry, ordered a chest X ray for comparison, and determined that an escalation of care and adjustment of medications was necessary. A complete blood count (CBC) with differential and basic metabolic panel was also ordered. While there was some reduction in oxygenation, it did not require the initiation of oxygen therapy, and the radiograph as reviewed (but not officially read by the treating clinician) did not show pneumonia. The treatment plan included the addition of an oral steroid medication prescribed along with the bronchodilator inhaler to account for the exacerbation in the patient's chronic conditions. The physician discussed hospitalization with the patient, and they determined that given his support at home, he could be managed as an outpatient if his condition responded to the treatment. The patient was then instructed to contact the medical office immediately or present to the emergency department if the inhaler and steroid combination failed to provide relief for the patient's acute symptoms, or in the event of any unwanted side effects, in order to further adjust the dosage as appropriate. Which MDM level(s) and E/M code(s) should be reported for this case study?

Case Study 3

A 12-year-old male established patient with attention deficit hyperactivity disorder (ADHD) presents for a follow-up visit for mild symptoms and minimal medication side effects. The patient is accompanied by his mother, and history is obtained from both. The patient reports that his grades are good but his appetite at lunch is poor. He eats well at other meals. His mother was told that he appears distracted in class. The physician reviews previous progress notes, plans to renew the patient's stimulant prescription with increased dosage, and advises the patient to return in two months for a follow-up visit. Which MDM level(s) and E/M code(s) should be reported for this case study?

Case Study 4

A 70-year-old female new patient presents to the office with her daughter, complaining of being depressed. Patient and daughter report increasing distress due to the patient repeatedly losing or misplacing small objects over the past several months. The patient has also noticed intermittent, mild forgetfulness of other people's names and what she intends to say during conversation, and the daughter confirms. No additional stressors are reported, although the patient reports mild sadness when thinking about her condition. The physician performs an appropriate neurologic examination and finds no remarkable findings beyond that the patient is unable to focus on the serial 7s and that she exhibits mild struggle with telling history. She remembers only one of three objects. The physician notes these findings in the medical record and, after shared decision making with the patient and her daughter, provides a prescription for a selective serotonin reuptake inhibitor for the patient's symptoms of depression, recommending a return visit and check-up in one month. The patient will also be evaluated by a specialist in neurology for impaired attention and declining memory; a referral is generated. Because dementia is thought to be a likely comorbidity, a CBC, vitamin B12 test, TSH test, and comprehensive metabolic panel are ordered. Which MDM level(s) and E/M code(s) should be reported for this case study?

Case Study 5

A 28-year-old male was brought to the urgent care clinic with a power-saw wound to his left palm. The patient was conscious but nauseated and was accompanied by his girlfriend. A targeted history was obtained and documented. The urgent care physician quickly evaluated him and ordered and interpreted a hand X ray (reported separately) to verify the apparent superficial depth of injury. The examination did not suggest significant tendon, nerve, or vascular injury. The physician advised that the wound would require layered closure with sutures. Which MDM level(s) and E/M code(s) should be reported for this case study?

Case Study 6

A carpenter presents to the office of his primary care physician complaining of swelling and erythema over the right index finger proximal interphalangeal (PIP) joint. He states that he removed a wood splinter from the finger a few days ago. Examination reveals fluctuance over the PIP joint combined with early lymphangitis that extends along the dorsal aspect of the long finger into the dorsum of the hand. Palpation of the palmar aspect of the PIP joint produces minimal discomfort. The patient is afebrile and has no adenopathy. Which MDM level(s) and E/M code(s) should be reported for this case study?

Case Study 7

A 58-year-old male who had a bileaflet mechanical prosthetic aortic valve replacement nine months ago is seen in the office with evidence of congestive heart failure secondary to aortic insufficiency. The physician reviews laboratory studies that reveal anemia secondary to hemolysis; there is no evidence of bacterial endocarditis. Cardiac catheterization studies performed a week ago are reviewed, revealing 4+ aortic insufficiency. A transesophageal echocardiogram performed the same day and independently interpreted (but not separately reported) by the physician reveals dehiscence of the valve in the area of the noncoronary cusp with motion of the prosthetic valve ring. The situation was discussed with the patient and his family, and he was scheduled for emergency surgery to repair the aortic valve. Which MDM level(s) and E/M code(s) should be reported for this case study?

Case Study 8

A 6-year-old male presents to the office with a history of snoring, mouth breathing, restless sleeping at night, and waking during the night. His parents describe periods of observed apnea for several seconds. He has some dysphagia for solid food and is often tired or cranky during the day. An audio recording of his breathing at night has been made. On physical examination, the child has 4+ enlarged tonsils. The physician orders a lateral neck radiograph. The report notes enlarged tonsils and adenoids. Which MDM level(s) and E/M code(s) should be reported for this case study?

Case Study 9

A 69-year-old male with hypertension and type 2 diabetes presents with sudden worsening of hearing in the left ear over a period of several days. He is found to have cerumen occluding the entire external auditory canal, which is amenable to removal by irrigation. The physician performs the procedure in the office. The hypertension and diabetes are not addressed during this visit and would not factor into the MDM determination. The performance of the procedure would not factor into the determination of the MDM for the visit. Which MDM level(s) and E/M code(s) should be reported for this case study?

Case Study 10

A 26-year-old female with a history of medical treatment for pelvic inflammatory disease presents to her gynecologist with right lower quadrant abdominal pain. The physician orders a beta human chorionic gonadotropin (HCG) test, CBC with differential, and pelvic ultrasound. Results indicate a beta HCG level of 4000, and the pelvic ultrasound findings are suggestive of an ectopic gestational sac in the proximal left fallopian tube or uterine cornua. The patient is scheduled for emergency surgery to treat the ectopic pregnancy. Which MDM level(s) and E/M code(s) should be reported for this case study?

SECTION 3

E/M 2021: Time and Code-Level Selection Changes

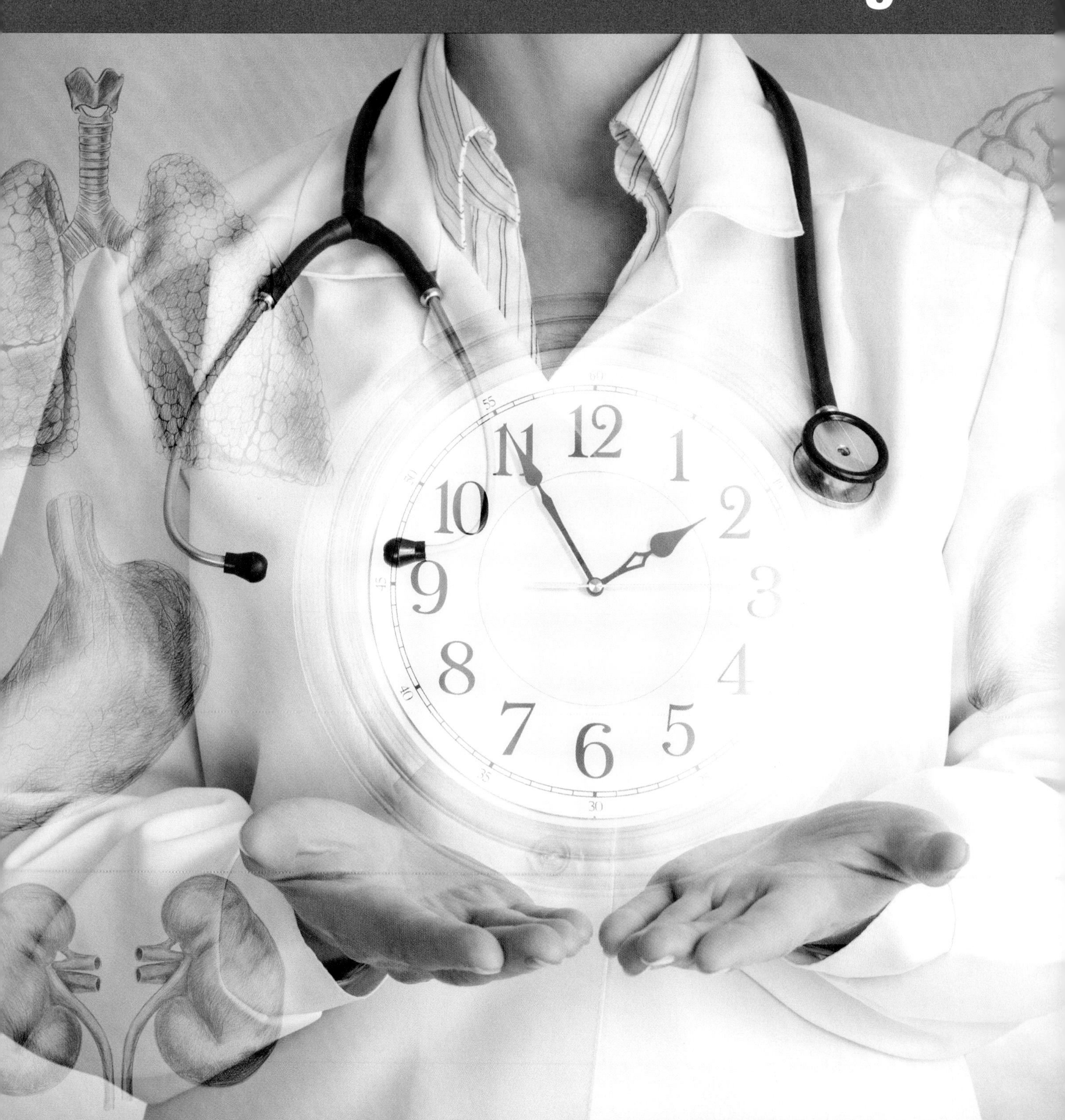

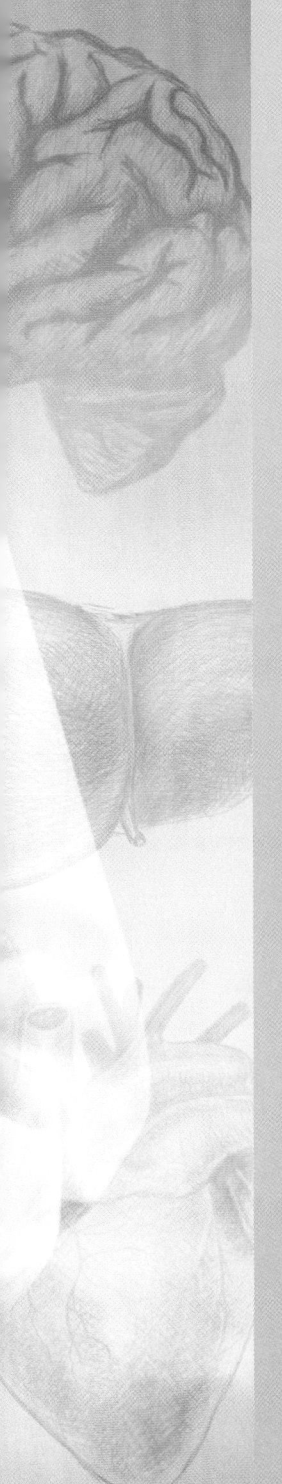

This section provides an overview of the reporting of time in the Current Procedural Terminology (CPT®) 2021 code set as a whole, an in-depth look at the changes implemented for reporting time for evaluation and management (E/M) office or other outpatient visits, and helpful reminders for the calculation of time in other E/M areas.

The objectives of this section are as follows:

- Examine how time has been represented in the CPT code set, specifically in E/M codes, since inception
- Review the changes for E/M office or other outpatient visit codes when using time as the criterion for code-level selection
- Compare time definitions across the range of E/M codes as of January 1, 2021
- Understand the impacts of the E/M changes for 2021 on other areas in the CPT code set

CHAPTER 3

Time

Overview

The CPT® code set contains many codes for which time is used as a basis for code selection. Many terms are used to describe time, reflecting the breadth and depth of the procedures and services represented. The different terms also reflect the multiple characteristics related to time that are key in understanding and quantifying the work performed (see Figure 1).

FIGURE 1 Distinct Time References in the CPT Code Set

Physician or Other Qualified Health Care Professional Time	Defining Time for a Component of Service Provided
Typical Face-to-face Non-face-to-face Clinical staff Bedside/floor/unit Approximate	Preservice Intraservice Postservice
Time Specific to a Procedure	**Extended Time Intervals**
Performance of a service Testing Documenting	Days Months

Along with the variation in terms, the instructions for how time is to be calculated are specified for each code type. Some codes have specific instructions for reporting time; in the absence of specific instructions, the broader CPT guidelines provide instructions for how time should be calculated. Examples of the broad CPT guidelines for reporting time include the instructions for reporting a unit of time when a single time value is specified within the code descriptor, and how to use the midpoint concept or the threshold concept to select the appropriate code when actual time falls between two typical times (see Figure 2).

FIGURE 2 Reporting Time per CPT Coding: Midpoints and Thresholds

The Midpoint Concept

A unit of time is attained when the midpoint is passed.

For example:
An hour is attained when 31 minutes have elapsed (more than midway between 0 and 60 minutes).

A second hour is attained when a total of 91 minutes have elapsed.

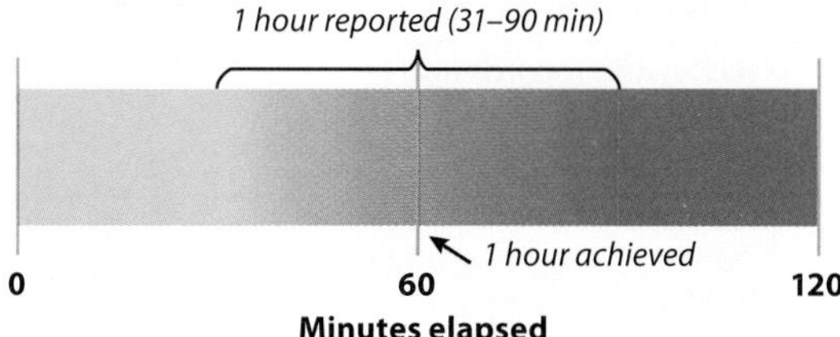

The Threshold Concept

When codes are ranked according to sequential typical times and the actual time is between two typical times, the code with the typical time closest to the actual time is used.

Use of Time in E/M Codes

The use of time in E/M codes has evolved over the years. Prior to 1992, time definitions for the levels of E/M services were implicit in the CPT code set. To add clarity and help define and select an appropriate level of E/M services, time was included as an explicit factor beginning with CPT 1992.

Surveys of practicing physicians were used to obtain data on the amount of time and work associated with typical E/M services. Physician work is defined by law as the time required to perform a particular service and the intensity of that service. The surveys showed relatively consistent times among specialties when describing total time for E/M services. Prior to 2021, the E/M office or other outpatient visit code selection was based on the level of history, physical examination, and medical decision making (MDM) involved in the encounter *unless* > 50% of the visit involved counseling and coordination of care. Face-to-face time with the patient and family could be used as a basis for code selection if > 50% of that visit was care coordination or counseling. The typical time within the code descriptor was used to select the appropriate code. (See Table 1.)

TABLE 1 Existing (Before 2021) E/M Office or Other Outpatient and Inpatient E/M Codes: Activities Included in Time and Work Calculation

		Office or Other Outpatient	Inpatient
Work of both components included in calculating the work of a typical service	Intraservice (focus for codes listing typical time)	**Face-to-face time:** Time spent with the patient and/or family Includes the time spent performing such tasks as obtaining a history, performing an examination, and counseling the patient	**Unit/floor time:** Time present on the patient's hospital unit and at the bedside rendering services for that patient. Includes the time to establish and/or review the patient's chart, examine the patient, write notes, and communicate with other professionals and the patient's family
	Pre- or postservice	**Non-face-to-face time:** Reviewing records and tests, arranging for further services, and communicating further with other professionals and the patient through written reports and telephone contact	Time spent off the patient's floor; tasks such as reviewing pathology and radiology findings in another part of the hospital

When time became an explicit component of the CPT code set in 1992, it was added to *assist* in selecting the most appropriate level of E/M service and not to *routinely supplant* the other components that define E/M services. These other components included key factors such as history, examination, and MDM and contributory factors such as counseling, coordination of care, and nature of the presenting problem.

Prior to the implementation of the 2021 CPT coding guidelines, the use of time as the determining factor to qualify for a particular level of E/M office or other outpatient service was permitted *only* when counseling and/or coordination of care dominated (ie, took up > 50% of the encounter). In addition, with regard to the type of care provided, only *face-to-face time* could be included in the time calculation.

Time Changes for E/M for 2021

The changes to E/M office or other outpatient codes, effective January 1, 2021, represent further evolutionary steps in the use and importance of time in code selection. The CPT and AMA/Specialty Society Relative Value Scale (RVS) Update Committee (RUC) E/M Workgroup focused on addressing two key concerns regarding documentation and code selection for office and other outpatient E/M codes: the need to increase flexibility and the need to decrease ambiguity in code selection.

Element Addressed: Increased Flexibility in Code Selection

Stakeholders expressed a need for greater flexibility in code selection to value the most relevant elements for a given patient encounter, recognizing that E/M services have changed substantially since the 1995 and 1997 documentation guidelines were published. The workgroup employed a series of surveys sent to a wide-ranging group of stakeholders to reach a consensus regarding the updated structure for 2021. As a result, for 2021, physicians and other qualified health care professionals (QHPs) have the option to select time or MDM to determine code selection. With the exception of code 99211, *time alone may be used to select the appropriate code level* for E/M office or other outpatient services (99202-99205, 99212-99215), whether or not counseling and/or coordination of care dominates the service. The definition of time has also been updated. It now includes the *total time* spent on the day of the encounter—not just face-to-face time with the patient and family. This is a significant change from prior definitions.

Element Addressed: Ambiguity

Before 2021, E/M office or other outpatient codes contained a single, typical time in the code descriptor. Because CPT guidelines mentioned both the use of midpoints and threshold values when choosing between two codes with typical times, it was not always clear to physicians, other QHPs, or coders what precise increment of time was needed to move to the next code level. In addition, there was often ambiguity regarding which elements of a visit could be included as part of the E/M typical time, which portions could be reported separately, and which were not to be individually identified as they were already incorporated in the pre- or postservice work components for a given code.

To address these ambiguities, the code descriptors have been changed to specify discrete, nonoverlapping time ranges for each code for 2021. These ranges represent total time on the day of the encounter, which includes both face-to-face and non-face-to-face time. Total time has replaced "typical" time (which represented face-to-face time) with the 2021 changes. This adjustment eliminates the need to employ midpoint and threshold values and provides concrete guidance when total time is employed as the key selection criterion. Note that time is unnecessary to qualify for the selection of code 99211 and, therefore, it has been removed as a selection criterion for that code effective January 1, 2021 (see Table 2).

ADVICE/ALERT NOTE

Total time must be documented in the health record when it is used as the basis for code selection. Third-party payers may have additional criteria regarding the acceptable level of documentation detail required when time is used for code selection, and they should be contacted to obtain their specific documentation requirements.

TABLE 2 CPT E/M Office or Other Outpatient Visits: Time Comparison

E/M Office or Other Outpatient Code	Typical Face-to-Face Time (Before 2021)	Total Time on the Day of the Encounter: Face-to-Face and Non-Face-to-Face Time* (2021)
New Patient		
99201	10 minutes	Code deleted
99202	20 minutes	15-29 minutes
99203	30 minutes	30-44 minutes
99204	45 minutes	45-59 minutes
99205	60 minutes	60-74 minutes
Established Patient		
99211	5 minutes	Time component removed
99212	10 minutes	10-19 minutes
99213	15 minutes	20-29 minutes
99214	25 minutes	30-39 minutes
99215	40 minutes	40-54 minutes

* Only on the date of the encounter. There are typical activities that take place before and after the date of the encounter that are not reported separately.

ADVICE/ALERT NOTE

Activities included in the calculation of total time for E/M office or other outpatient codes in 2021 include both face-to-face and non-face-to-face activities.

Time Calculation: Activities Included

Before 2021, some of the non-face-to-face activities may have been included in the pre- or post-visit work, but the time spent on them was not included in the calculation of typical time. The changes bring additional clarity on how and when these aspects of a service should be reported. Activities reported separately are not to be included in the calculation of total time.

For the 2021 E/M office or other outpatient changes, the total time spent by the physician or other QHP on the day of the encounter may include the activities listed in Table 3. Note that the list includes both face-to-face and non-face-to-face activities.

TABLE 3 E/M Office or Other Outpatient Codes in 2021: Sample List of Included Activities in Calculation of Total Time

Activity(ies)	Primarily Face-to-Face?
Preparing to see the patient (eg, review of tests)	No
Obtaining and/or reviewing separately obtained history	No
Performing a medically appropriate examination and/or evaluation	Yes
Counseling and educating the patient/family/caregiver	Yes
Ordering medications, tests, or procedures	No
Referring to and communicating with other health care professionals (when not separately reported)	No
Documenting clinical information in the electronic or other health record	No
Independently interpreting results (not separately reported)	No
Communicating results to the patient/family/caregiver	No
Care coordination (not separately reported)	No

Code Selection vs Code Valuation: Pre- and Post-Visit Changes

The survey methodology utilized by RUC for quantifying the work associated with the E/M office or other outpatient codes prior to 2021 categorized certain non-face-to-face activities—on the day of the encounter as well as on the dates prior to or following the date of the encounter—as pre- or postservice. The intraservice time included *only* face-to-face encounter time, designated as the typical time. The activities performed before and after the face-to-face encounter were not used to determine typical time (which was defined as intraservice time), but they were included in the work estimate for that code.

For the E/M office or other outpatient codes that have been revised for 2021, while the total time on the date of the encounter determines the code to be selected, the work value for the code, as determined by the RUC surveys completed for the 2021 revisions, is based on the entire time spent by the physician from 3 days before the visit to 7 days after the visit. The time ranges in the code descriptors define the intraservice times for these encounters (total time on the day of the encounter), while the time spent in typical activities during the 3 days before and 7 days after the visit accounts for the preservice and postservice times and work.

RUC approved the use of 3 days prior to and 7 days following the office visits based on instructions within the CPT guidelines of not reporting certain non-face-to-face services that relate to work performed before or after the office visit (eg, telephone services and interprofessional consultations). It is important to remember this distinction when evaluating a pre- or postservice activity completed on a date other than the date of the encounter. For example, the communication of test results a few days after the date of the encounter should not be reported separately because the work and time of that communication has already been incorporated into the valuation of the office visit (see Figure 3).

FIGURE 3 E/M Office or Other Outpatient Codes: Work Considered for Code Valuation vs Time Reported for Code Selection

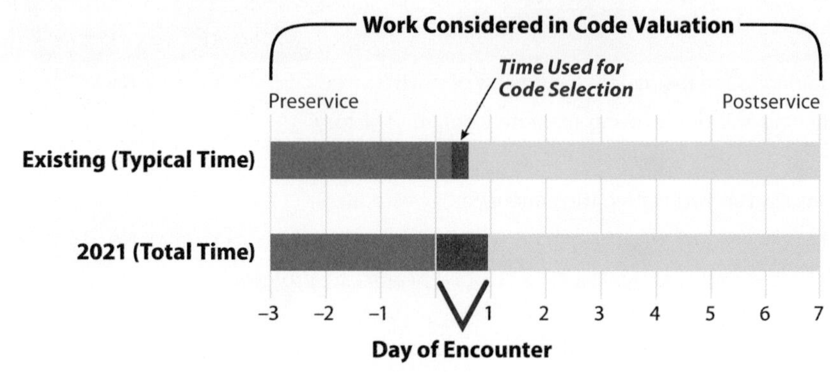

Code-Selection Methodology: Time or MDM

Because either MDM or total time on the day of the encounter may be used to choose the appropriate level of E/M service for office and other outpatient visit codes, coders and practice managers—as well as physicians and other QHPs—have asked whether one method of reporting is more advantageous than the other. The methodology that incorporates the most appropriate and relevant elements for a given patient encounter should be used.

The choice to select a code level based on time or MDM will vary with the presenting concerns of the patient and the time and complexity of the encounter. The E/M guidelines for office or other outpatient visits do not describe an advantage of either MDM or time; rather, the determination should reflect the time and intensity of the service provided. The choice depends entirely on the nature of the visit. High-acuity short visits will likely be reported using MDM as the criterion, whereas prolonged, time-intensive visits may be better reported using total time on the date of the encounter.

Clinical Staff Time and E/M Code Selection

The CPT code set defines a clinical staff member as “a person who works under the supervision of a physician or other qualified health care professional, and who is allowed by law, regulation and facility policy to perform or assist in the performance of a specified professional service, but does not individually report that professional service.” Time spent by clinical staff may not be included in the calculation of total time for the purposes of code selection when the physician or other QHP performs the face-to-face services of the encounter. Clinical staff time is included in the practice expense component of the total RVUs allocated for that code.

When code 99211 is used, time should not be used for code selection. For this code—*Office or other outpatient visit for the evaluation and management of an established patient, that may not require the presence of a physician or other qualified health care professional. Usually, the presenting problem(s) are minimal*—the physician's or other QHP's time is spent supervising clinical staff who actually performs the face-to-face service rather than performing the work himself or herself. Note that the time component has been removed from this code for 2021.

Time Calculation of Shared or Split Visits: Distinct Time

A shared or split visit is defined in the CPT 2021 E/M guidelines as a visit in which a physician and other QHP(s) jointly provide the face-to-face and non-face-to-face work related to the visit. When time is used to select the appropriate level of service, the time personally spent by both the physician and other QHP(s) for the E/M service on the date of the encounter is summed to define total time. Only the distinct individual time of each person should be summed for shared or split visits; if both individuals jointly meet with or discuss the patient, only the time of one individual should be counted. See the following example.

EXAMPLE

Shared or Split E/M Visits: Time Calculation Example

Dr W and physician assistant (PA) S both spent time seeing Mrs J, an established patient, for an E/M office visit. Dr W spent a total of **25 minutes** on the day of service. PA S spent a total of **18 minutes** on the day of service. Time for both the physician and the PA includes **8 minutes spent jointly meeting** with Mrs J.

The total time to be reported on the day of service is **25 + 18 – 8 = 35 minutes.**

The 8 minutes spent meeting jointly with the patient should be counted for only one individual.

Definitions of Time Across E/M Code Groups

Although the guidelines for calculation of time for E/M office or other outpatient visit codes have changed substantially in the CPT 2021 code set, the changes are effective *only* for E/M codes 99202-99205 and 99211-99215; definitions for time calculation have not changed for other E/M service codes. Make sure to use the appropriate definition of time (ie, office or other outpatient E/M visits vs all other E/M visits) when reporting a given E/M service. A summary of time definitions, as well as activities that should be included in time calculation for coding purposes by E/M code group, is provided in Table 4.

TABLE 4 E/M Code Category: Time Calculations for 2021

E/M Code Category	Definition of Time for Coding Purposes	Activities Included in Time Calculation
Office or Other Outpatient (99202-99205, 99212-99215)	Total time on date of encounter personally spent by the physician and/or other QHP includes face-to-face and non-face-to-face time	• Preparing to see the patient (eg, review of tests) • Obtaining and/or reviewing separately obtained history • Performing a medically appropriate examination and/or evaluation • Counseling and educating the patient, family, and/or caregiver • Ordering medications, tests, or procedures • Referring and communicating with other health care professionals (when not separately reported) • Documenting clinical information in the electronic or other health record • Care coordination (not separately reported) • Independently interpreting results (not separately reported) and communicating results to the patient, family, and/or caregiver
Office or Other Outpatient Consultations (99241-99245); Domiciliary, Rest Home (eg, Boarding Home), or Custodial Care Services (99324-99328, 99334-99337); Home Services (99341-99345, 99347-99350); Cognitive Assessment and Care Plan Services (99483)	Face-to-face time with the patient and/or family	• Face-to-face time with the patient and/or family • Obtaining history • Examining the patient • Counseling the patient
Hospital Observation Services (99218-99220, 99224-99226, 99234-99236); Hospital Inpatient Services (99221-99223, 99231-99233); Inpatient Consultations (99251-99255); Nursing Facility Services (99304-99318)	Unit/floor time that includes the time present on the patient's hospital unit and at the bedside rendering services for that patient	• Establishing and/or reviewing the patient's chart • Examining the patient • Writing notes • Communicating with other professionals and the patient's family Note: Time is not a descriptive component for E/M levels of emergency department services.

Time definitions and methods for determining the appropriate code level for all categories of E/M codes are provided in Table 5. Because typical time measures are still used in other E/M code groups, it is essential to refer to the unique guidelines for each category of E/M service, particularly regarding the use of threshold values and midpoints, in order to use the appropriate method for code selection.

TABLE 5 Measuring and Reporting Time For E/M Codes *(Changes Effective January 1, 2021)*

Category	Subcategory(ies)	CPT Codes	Reported Time
Office or Other Outpatient Services			
	New Patient	**99202-99205**	Total (on day of encounter)
	Established Patient	**99212-99215**	Total (on day of encounter)
Hospital Observation Services			
	Observation Care Discharge Services	**99217**	N/A
	Initial Observation Care	**99218-99220**	Typical
	Subsequent Observation Care	**99224-99226**	Typical
Hospital Inpatient Services			
	Initial Hospital Care	**99221-99223**	Typical
	Subsequent Hospital Care	**99231-99233**	Typical
	Hospital Discharge Services	**99238, 99239**	Total time spent on discharge
Observation or Inpatient Care Services (Including Admission and Discharge Services)		**99234-99236**	Typical
Consultations			
	Office or Other Outpatient	**99241-99245**	Typical
	Inpatient	**99251-99255**	Typical
Emergency Department Services			
	New or Established Patient	**99281-99285**	N/A
	Other Emergency Services	**99288**	N/A
Critical Care Services			
	Time-based Critical Care	**99291, 99292**	Specified interval
Nursing Facility Services			
	Initial Nursing Facility Care	**99304-99306**	Typical
	Subsequent Nursing Facility Care	**99307-99310**	Typical
	Nursing Facility Discharge Services	**99315, 99316**	Specified interval
	Other Nursing Facility Services	**99318**	Typical
Domiciliary, Rest Home (eg, Boarding Home), or Custodial Care Services			
	New Patient	**99324-99328**	Typical
	Established Patient	**99334-99337**	Typical
Domiciliary, Rest Home (eg, Assisted Living Facility), or Home Care Plan Oversight Services		**99339, 99340**	Specified interval
Home Services			
	New Patient	**99341-99345**	Typical
	Established Patient	**99347-99350**	Typical
Preventive Medicine Services			
	New Patient	**99381-99387**	N/A
	Established Patient	**99391-99397**	N/A
	Preventive Medicine, Individual Counseling	**99401-99404**	Approximate

(continued)

TABLE 5 Measuring and Reporting Time For E/M Codes *(Changes Effective January 1, 2021), continued*

Category	Subcategory(ies)	CPT Codes	Reported Time
Preventive Medicine Services, *continued*			
	Behavior Change Interventions, Individual	**99406-99409**	Specified interval
	Preventive Medicine, Group Counseling	**99411, 99412**	Specified interval
	Unlisted Preventive Medicine Services	**99429**	N/A
Non-Face-to-Face Services			
	Telephone Services	**99441-99443**	Specified interval
	Online Digital Evaluation and Management Services	**99421-99423**	Specified interval
	Interprofessional Telephone/Internet/Electronic Health Record Consultations	**99446-99449, 99451, 99452**	Specified interval
	Digitally Stored Data Services/Remote Physiologic Monitoring	**99453, 99454, 99091, 99473, 99474**	N/A (99453) or per 30-day period
	Remote Physiologic Monitoring Treatment Management Services	**99457-99458**	Per 30-day period
Special Evaluation and Management Services			
	Basic Life and/or Disability Evaluation Services	**99450**	N/A
	Work Related or Medical Disability Evaluation Services	**99455, 99456**	N/A
Newborn Care Services		**99460-99463**	Per day
Delivery/Birthing Room Attendance and Resuscitation Services		**99464, 99465**	N/A
Inpatient Neonatal Intensive Care Services and Pediatric and Neonatal Critical Care Services			
	Pediatric Critical Care Patient Transport	**99466, 99467, 99485, 99486**	Specified interval
	Inpatient Neonatal and Pediatric Critical Care	**99468-99476**	Per day
	Initial and Continuing Intensive Care Services	**99477-99480**	Per day
Cognitive Assessment and Care Plan Services		**99483**	Typical
Care Management Services			
	Chronic Care Management Services	**99490, 99491**	Interval per calendar month
	Complex Chronic Management Services	**99487-99489**	Specified interval
Psychiatric Collaborative Care Management Services		**99492-99494**	Interval per calendar month
Transitional Care Management Services		**99495, 99496**	N/A
Advance Care Planning		**99497, 99498**	Specified interval
General Behavioral Health Integration Care Management		**99484**	Interval per calendar month
Other Evaluation and Management Services		**99499**	N/A

Considerations When Using Other CPT Codes or Modifiers

The E/M office or other outpatient visit changes for 2021 will naturally have some effects on other E/M codes and/or CPT modifiers, which will require some considerations when and if they are used. This is discussed in the following sections.

Considerations When Using Other E/M Codes

The 2021 changes also affect some other codes within the E/M section of the CPT 2021 code set. The principal changes are outlined in Table 6.

TABLE 6 Effects of New Code 99417 on Other E/M Codes

Codes	E/M Category	Effect
#★+●**99417**	Prolonged Service With or Without Direct Patient Contact on the Date of an Office or Other Outpatient Service	Addition of new shorter prolonged services add-on code; to be used only with **99205** and **99215** when time is chosen as the method for selecting code level
★+▲**99354** ★+▲**99355** +▲**99356** +**99357**	Prolonged Service With Direct Patient Contact	Revised descriptor No longer used with **99202-99205, 99212-99215**
99358 +**99359**	Prolonged Service Without Direct Patient Contact	Revised descriptor No longer used with **99202-99205, 99212-99215** on the day of service. May be reported on subsequent days *if* the service is beyond the designated postservice work of the encounter
99366-99368	Case Management Services Medical Team Conferences	Time (calculation); any time reported with **99366-99368** may not be considered in the total time for reporting **99202-99215**
#+▲**99415** #+▲**99416**	Prolonged Clinical Staff Services With Physician or Other Qualified Health Care Professional Supervision	Revised descriptor Time (calculation); begins beyond highest time in range of base code versus typical time

Changes in the E/M section primarily affect the E/M office or other outpatient services and prolonged services guidelines and codes. The remaining E/M guidelines and codes have not changed. The following distinctions should also be noted:

- For prolonged services, there is a shorter prolonged services code to capture each 15 minutes of medically necessary physician or other QHP work beyond the time captured by the office or other outpatient service E/M code; it is used only when the office or other outpatient code is selected using total time. Prolonged services of less than 15 minutes should not be reported.
- Time calculation affects the reporting of prolonged services and the reporting of case management services by medical teams, because time is calculated based on the *total* physician or other QHP time spent on the date of the encounter. Total time includes both face-to-face and non-face-to-face services. Clear, nonoverlapping time ranges have been included in each code descriptor (see the following example).

Time

EXAMPLE

E/M Service With Case Management

Mr J, a 55-year-old established patient with rheumatoid arthritis, hypertension, hyperlipidemia, and type 2 diabetes mellitus with neuropathy, presents for a follow-up office visit, complaining of tiredness and heightened stress levels brought about by increased work hours over the past 2 months. Dr S, a family practice physician, reviews the medical history form and vital signs obtained by clinical staff; a medically appropriate history and examination, are performed. Dr S discusses potential diagnoses and treatment options including stress reduction techniques with the patient. A total time of 23 minutes is spent prior to and during the patient encounter.

Later that same day, Dr S meets for an extended conference with three other physicians directly involved with Mr Jones' care: Dr A, a cardiologist who saw Mr J last week; Dr C, an endocrinologist who saw Mr J 2 weeks ago, and Dr Williams, a rheumatologist who saw Mr J last month. Together, they review Mr J's medical record and their individual assessments of his condition, devising an optimal care plan in a coordinated manner given the multiple domains requiring attention (biomedical, psychological, and functional). The conference lasts 35 minutes.

Later that evening, Dr S spends an additional 10 minutes completing documentation, of which 6 minutes consisted of record keeping and report generation pertaining to the team conference.

The total time spent by Dr S on the day of the encounter pertaining to Mr J's care is 68 minutes; however, time reported for medical team conferences may not be used in the determination of time for other services, including any E/M service.

Given the reporting guideline above, the following codes should be reported:

Report code 99367, *Medical team conference with interdisciplinary team of health care professionals, patient and/or family not present, 30 minutes or more; participation by physician,* for the medical team conference, reflecting the 35 minutes spent in the conference. The 6 minutes of record keeping and report generation pertaining to the team conference are not counted separately.

Report E/M code 99213 for the office visit when reporting on the basis of total time; the remaining 27 minutes (68 minutes – 35 minutes for the team conference – 6 minutes not separately reported) spent on the day of the encounter (23 minutes of face-to-face time + 4 minutes of non-face-to-face time) would be the total time assigned to the office visit.

Additional information on the 2021 changes in prolonged services codes will be discussed in Section 4 of this book.

Considerations When Using E/M With Other Services and Procedures

The 2021 changes in the E/M section do not affect most other sections of the CPT code set; however, certain guidelines for the reporting of E/M office or other outpatient codes together with other services should be reviewed to ensure proper reporting.

E/M Office or Other Outpatient Services With a Procedure

As stated in the overall CPT guidelines, when another service is performed concurrently with a time-based service, the time associated with the concurrent service should not be included in the time used for reporting the time-based service. E/M office or other outpatient visits will incorporate total time on the date of the encounter as an available selection criterion. When total time is used for code selection, be sure that the time associated with activities used to meet criteria for the E/M service does not overlap with the time required to perform a procedure on the same day, particularly with non-face-to-face activities.

Psychotherapy Codes for E/M Services

In the Psychotherapy subsection of the Medicine section, the guidelines state that add-on codes 90833, 90836, and 90838 may be used with E/M codes if E/M services are provided with psychotherapy services. The guidelines give specific instructions regarding how time is calculated and used. Per the guidelines, time associated with activities used to meet criteria for the E/M service is not included in the time used for reporting the psychotherapy service (ie, time spent on history, examination, and MDM). The time required to provide the E/M service is not counted toward the psychotherapy time. *Time may not be used as the basis for E/M code selection* and prolonged services may not be reported when psychotherapy services (90833, 90836, 90838) are reported with E/M codes.

Use of E/M-Focused Modifiers

There are four key E/M-related modifiers: 24, 25, 57, and 95 (see Table 7).

TABLE 7 E/M-Focused Modifiers

Modifier	Descriptor
24	Unrelated Evaluation and Management Service by the Same Physician or Other Qualified Health Care Professional During a Postoperative Period
25	Significant, Separately Identifiable Evaluation and Management Service by the Same Physician or Other Qualified Health Care Professional on the Same Day of the Procedure or Other Service
57	Decision for Surgery
95	Synchronous Telemedicine Service Rendered via a Real-Time Interactive Audio and Video Telecommunications System

ADVICE/ALERT NOTE

The CPT 2021 E/M service guidelines have been revised to include guidelines common to all E/M services, as well as specific guidelines for office or other outpatient services and for other E/M services. Review the instructions for each category or subcategory of E/M services to ensure appropriate code selection.

Modifier-specific considerations are outlined below. Note that the modifiers reviewed here cannot be used with E/M code 99211 because that service is performed by clinical staff, and the presence of the physician or other QHP is not required.

Modifier 24: Unrelated Evaluation and Management Service by the Same Physician or Other Qualified Health Care Professional During a Postoperative Period

Use of this modifier will not change in 2021. If total time is used to determine the E/M code selected, ensure that the time spent on activities for the E/M service, particularly non-face-to-face activities, does not overlap with any of the services relating to the postoperative period.

Modifier 25: Significant, Separately Identifiable Evaluation and Management Service by the Same Physician or Other Qualified Health Care Professional on the Same Day of the Procedure or Other Service

This modifier reflects a significant, separately identifiable E/M service on the same day as a procedure or other service. It is important to avoid double-counting time or activities that overlap between the E/M service and the procedure or other service. The need to differentiate is particularly important when the E/M service is prompted by the symptom or condition for which the procedure and/or service was provided. This is not a change from current coding guidelines.

Modifier 57: Decision for Surgery

No changes are expected with this modifier.

Modifier 95: Synchronous Telemedicine Service Rendered via a Real-Time Interactive Audio and Video Telecommunications System

Appendix A of the CPT 2020 code set notes that the totality of the communication of information exchanged between the physician or other QHP and the patient during the course of the synchronous telemedicine service must be of an amount and nature that would be sufficient to meet the key components and/or requirements of the same service when rendered via a face-to-face interaction. It is not yet clear how these criteria will be interpreted by third-party payers when total time on the day of encounter is used for code selection; specifically, it is not clear how payers will respond to incorporation of the time required to perform non-face-to-face activities that do not involve the patient directly.

Evaluate Your Understanding

The following questions and case studies are critical checkpoints that are meant to let you apply your critical thinking and evaluate your understanding of the content covered in the chapter. The answers for the end-of-chapter exercises are available at amaproductupdates.org.

A Multiple Choice Questions

Select the correct or most appropriate answer(s) to the following questions.

1. Which of these is seen as an objective, verifiable measure that correlates with physicians' work estimates?
   a. MDM
   b. Time
   c. Documentation
   d. Coordination of care

2. Which of these refers to a segment of an encounter that often appeared as the "typical time" before 2021?
   a. Intraservice time
   b. Preservice time
   c. Postservice time
   d. Non-face-to-face time

3. Which of these best describes the midpoint concept?
   a. Each code has a discrete, nonoverlapping time range.
   b. A physician and other qualified health care professional(s) jointly provide the face-to-face and non-face-to-face work related to a visit.
   c. When codes are ranked according to sequential typical times and the actual time is between two typical times, the code with the typical time closest to the actual time is used.
   d. A certain unit of time is attained only when the midpoint of that time is met; for example, an hour is attained when 31 minutes have elapsed.

4. Which of these best describes the threshold concept?
   a. Each code has a discrete, nonoverlapping time range.
   b. A physician and other qualified health care professional(s) jointly provide the face-to-face and non-face-to-face work related to a visit.
   c. When codes are ranked according to sequential typical times and the actual time is between two typical times, the code with the typical time closest to the actual time is used.
   d. A certain unit of time is attained only when the midpoint of that time is met; for example, an hour is attained when 31 minutes have elapsed.

5. In the CPT code set, which of these terms refers to a person who works under the supervision of a physician or other qualified health care professional and is allowed by law, regulation, and facility policy to perform or assist in the performance of a specified professional service, but does not individually report that professional service?
   a. Clinical staff
   b. Receptionist
   c. Physician assistant
   d. Practice manager

6. Which of these would be considered a shared or split visit?
   a. A physician provides a synchronous telemedicine service.
   b. A physician or other qualified health care professional communicates test results to the patient and the patient's family.
   c. A physician refers a patient to another qualified health care professional.
   d. A physician and another qualified health care professional jointly provide the face-to-face and non-face-to-face work related to a visit.

7. Which of the following is the definition of modifier 24?
   a. Significant, Separately Identifiable Evaluation and Management Service by the Same Physician or Other Qualified Health Care Professional on the Same Day of the Procedure or Other Service.
   b. Synchronous Telemedicine Service Rendered via a Real-Time Interactive Audio and Video Telecommunications System.
   c. Decision for Surgery.
   d. Unrelated Evaluation and Management Service by the Same Physician or Other Qualified Health Care Professional During a Postoperative Period.

8. Significant, Separately Identifiable Evaluation and Management Service by the Same Physician or Other Qualified Health Care Professional on the Same Day of the Procedure or Other Service is the definition of which modifier?
   a. Modifier 22
   b. Modifier 57
   c. Modifier 25
   d. None of the above

9. Which of the following is the definition of modifier 57?
   a. Significant, Separately Identifiable Evaluation and Management Service by the Same Physician or Other Qualified Health Care Professional on the Same Day of the Procedure or Other Service.
   b. Synchronous Telemedicine Service Rendered via a Real-Time Interactive Audio and Video Telecommunications System.
   c. Decision for Surgery.
   d. Unrelated Evaluation and Management Service by the Same Physician or Other Qualified Health Care Professional During a Postoperative Period.

10. Synchronous Telemedicine Service Rendered via a Real-Time Interactive Audio and Video Telecommunications System is the definition of which modifier?
   a. Modifier 57
   b. Modifier 25
   c. Modifier 95
   d. None of the above

Time

B True/False Questions

Answer true (T) or false (F) to the following statements.

1. ______ Except for code 99211, time alone may be used to select the appropriate level of code for office or other outpatient E/M services.

2. ______ For codes 99202-99205 and 99212-99215, total time on the date of the encounter personally spent by the physician and/or other QHP includes face-to-face and non-face-to-face time.

3. ______ The 2021 office or other outpatient E/M coding changes indicate that calculation of the total time spent by the physician or other QHP on the day of the encounter may include the following activity as an example: documenting clinical information in the electronic or other health record.

4. ______ For codes 99202-99205 and 99212-99215, time will be calculated as typical time on the date of the encounter personally spent by the physician and/or other QHP.

5. ______ Unit/floor time does not include time present at the patient's bedside rendering services for the patient.

6. ______ In 2021, total time for code 99215 is 40-54 minutes.

7. ______ In 2021, definitions for time calculation will not change for E/M services other than services represented by codes 99202-99205 and 99212-99215.

8. ______ Time ranges specified in each code descriptor are discrete and nonoverlapping, providing concrete guidance when total time is employed as the key selection criterion.

9. ______ Clinical staff time is not included in the practice expense calculation.

10. ______ Time must be documented in the medical record when it is used as the basis for code selection.

11. ______ When time is used to select the appropriate level of service and when time-based reporting of a split or shared visit is allowed, the time personally spent by the physician and/or other QHP for the E/M service on the date of the encounter is summed to define total time.

12. ______ When split or shared visits are reported, if both health care professionals are jointly meeting with or discussing the patient, only the time of one individual should be counted.

C Fill in the Blank

Fill in the blank in the following statements with the most correct response.

1. Time is to be calculated for codes 99202-99205 and 99212-99215 based on ______________ the date of the encounter, including both the face-to-face and non-face-to-face time personally spent by the physician and/or other QHP.
2. Time spent by ______________ may not be included in the calculation of total time for the purposes of code selection when the physician or other QHP performs the face-to-face services of the encounter.
3. ______________ time includes the time present on the patient's hospital unit and at the bedside rendering services for that patient.
4. Only the distinct individual time of each person should be summed for ______________ visits; if both are jointly meeting with or discussing the patient, only the time of one individual should be counted.
5. For codes other than those for office or other outpatient services, a unit of time is attained when the ______________ is passed.
6. Total time includes both ______________ and non-face-to-face services.
7. The modifiers reviewed in this section may not be used with E/M code ______________ when that service is performed by nonclinical staff.
8. Emergency department codes are not ______________ dependent for code selection.
9. Prolonged services will be reported only with the ______________ time ranges (99205 or 99215) and only when ______________ is the basis for code selection.
10. In the Medicine/Psychotherapy subsection, activities used to meet criteria for the E/M service are not included in the time used for reporting the ______________.
11. The communication of information exchanged between the physician or other QHP and the patient during the course of synchronous ______________ must be of an amount and nature that would be sufficient to meet the key components and/or requirements of the same service when rendered via a face-to-face interaction.

D Internet-based Exercises 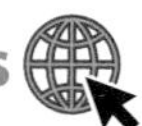

1. For more information to help you grasp the future roles of time and MDM for accurate coding, check out https://blog.supercoder.com/coding-updates/e-m-2021-grasp-the-future-roles-of-time-and-mdm-for-accurate-coding/.
2. To see how the 2021 E/M changes will affect your practice, visit https://www.icd10monitor.com/e-m-changes-how-will-they-affect-your-practice.
3. To read more about the 2021 E/M guideline and leveling changes, visit https://www.physicianspractice.com/view/2021-e-m-guideline-and-leveling-changes.
4. For additional quizzes about the E/M 2021 changes, visit https://quizlet.com/516959859/evaluation-and-management-changes-2021-diagram/.
5. For an online course about the E/M Coding Update, visit https://emuniversity.com/2021.html.

Time

E Short Answer Questions

Answer the following questions with the most correct response.

1. In 2021, for the selection of office or other outpatient E/M codes, are time and counseling/coordination of care both needed to determine the level of service?
2. In 2020, only face-to-face time is included in the time calculation for office or other outpatient E/M codes when it is used for code selection. Is this guideline the same in 2021?
3. In 2021, is the ordering of medications, tests, or procedures counted toward the calculation of the total time spent by the physician or other QHP on the day of the encounter for office or other outpatient services?
4. With the deletion of code 99201 in 2021, does this mean that services less than 15 minutes can no longer be reported for new patients?
5. A clinical staff member assists the physician during the patient's visit. Can the physician add this time to the physician's own time when determining the appropriate level of service?
6. The physician and the QHP both provide services to the patient during an encounter, but at different times. How is the time calculated?
7. If the physician and the QHP jointly provide services to the patient during an encounter, how is the time calculated?
8. If a physician spends 5 minutes with a patient and then is joined by the physician assistant (PA) and they spend aother 3 minutes jointly with the patient, after which the physician leaves and the PA spends another 20 minutes with the patient, how is the reportable time counted according to the rules for split or shared visits?
9. Is it necessary to document time when it is used for code selection?
10. Will all E/M codes be affected by the new guidelines for calculation of time for E/M codes?
11. Code 99211 has no time associated with it. Is this an error?
12. We typically report code 99201 for an initial office visit to remove sutures placed by another physician for a simple wound. How would this service be reported in 2021?

Time

F Case Studies

Although each of the following scenarios may involve service(s) or procedure(s) besides E/M, code only the E/M services. Use the *CPT 2021* codebook to determine the correct code(s) to report the E/M service(s) associated with each of the following procedure(s) or service(s).

Case Study 1

Dr R sees a 20-year-old established patient for an office visit. The patient presents with complaints consistent with an upper respiratory tract infection (URTI). The physician reviews the medical history form completed by the patient and vital signs obtained by a medical assistant. A history (including response to treatment at last visit and review of old medical records) and a relevant examination are performed. Dr R confirms the straightforward URTI diagnosis. The patient asks for a prescription for antibiotics, and Dr R spends considerable time explaining current guidelines for management of uncomplicated URTIs and the serious consequences of antibiotic overuse. A progress note is then completed by the physician. Dr R spent 21 minutes performing patient activities. Using time, which E/M code(s) should be reported for this case study?

Case Study 2

A 63-year-old female new patient with hypertension presents for a primary care visit after moving to the area. Blood pressure is adequately controlled with medication. Dr W reviews the medical history form completed by the patient and vital signs obtained by the medical assistant. The diagnosis of hypertension is confirmed with no new conditions identified. Time is spent discussing the ongoing treatment with the patient, including options for lifestyle modification, instructions to continue the current medication, and a discussion of preventive health care needs. A prescription is written to refill the current medication, with further discussion about joining Dr W's practice for ongoing primary care. A progress note is dictated after the encounter. Dr W spends 42 minutes performing patient activities. Using time as the basis for code selection, which E/M code(s) should be reported for this case study?

Case Study 3

A 45-year-old established patient with rheumatoid arthritis, hypertension, and hyperlipidemia presents for an office visit. His joint disease has been stable in the past, but in the last three weeks he has noticed increasing pain and has developed redness in several joints. He has had a low-grade fever for the past week. The evening before the visit, Dr J reviews the patient's recent test results for 15 minutes. At the visit, Dr J reviews the medical history form completed by the patient and vital signs obtained by the medical assistant. A history including prior response to treatment, a review of interval correspondence with other providers, and a relevant examination are performed. The likely progression of disease is discussed with the patient. Lab work to rule out systemic infection is ordered. A treatment plan is updated with a new medication prescription provided. The patient has considerable anxiety regarding the new medication and the potential risks, and Dr J provides additional information and counseling. Appropriate medical record documentation is made with a notation to follow up on the lab work results and to revise the treatment plan, as necessary. Dr J spends a total of 60 minutes in face-to-face and non-face-to-face activities relating to the visit. Using time as the basis for code selection, which E/M code(s) should be reported for this case study?

Case Study 4

A 60-year-old female new patient presents for an office visit. She complains of heart palpitations with occasional dizziness. The medical history form completed by the patient and vital signs obtained by clinical staff are reviewed. Dr I obtains a relevant history, performs an appropriate examination, orders an EKG, and reviews the medical data from other specialists the patient has seen within the multispecialty group practice. Dr I queries the patient about recent life events that may be impacting her health and discusses potential diagnoses with the patient and her family. Necessary lab work is arranged. There is extensive discussion with the patient about the recent death of her long-term partner and the possible impact on her current symptoms. The medical record is documented with a notation to check the results of the scheduled EKG and lab work and to revise treatment plan(s) as necessary. Dr I spends a total of 58 minutes on the date of the encounter. Using time as the basis for code selection, which E/M code(s) should be reported for this case study?

Case Study 5

A 55-year-old established patient with a history of hypertension and hyperlipidemia presents for a follow-up office visit. Dr T reviews recent test results and vital signs obtained by clinical staff. An appropriate history (including response to treatment at last visit) is obtained, and a medically appropriate examination is performed. Dr T discusses the plan and continuation of current medication with the patient, and refills current medications. Notations are made in the medical record. No additional testing is needed at this time. A total time of 22 minutes is spent on the date of the encounter. Using time as the basis for code selection, which E/M code(s) should be reported for this case study?

Case Study 6

A 42-year-old female new patient presents with a rash consistent with poison ivy that is not responding to over-the-counter medications. Dr W reviews the medical history form completed by the patient and vital signs obtained by clinical staff; obtains a medically appropriate history, including past rashes and allergy history; and performs a physical examination of the affected areas of the skin. Dr W discusses diagnosis, treatment options, and preventive health care needs with the patient. A new prescription is written. A total of 15 minutes is spent on the date of the encounter. Using time as the basis for code selection, which E/M code(s) should be reported for this case study?

Case Study 7

A 63-year-old male new patient comes in with a history of type 2 diabetes mellitus, coronary artery disease, osteoarthritis, chronic bronchitis, hypertension, gastroesophageal reflux, and hyperlipidemia. He presents with a 20-pound weight loss, dysphagia, and abdominal pain. He is on multiple medications and has not seen a physician for 18 months. Dr J reviews the medical history form completed by the patient and vital signs obtained by clinical staff, obtains a history, reviews outside medical records, and performs a medically appropriate examination. Dr J discusses potential diagnoses, treatment options, and preventive health care needs with the patient. The next day, Dr J completes a 5-minute telephone conversation with the patient's previous primary care physician and spends an additional 12 minutes completing the comprehensive treatment plan. A total time of 79 total minutes is spent on the encounter. Using time as the basis for code selection, which E/M code(s) should be reported for this case study?

Case Study 8

Dr A sees an established 3-year-old female patient with a two-day history of ear pain, fever, cough, and inability to sleep at night. Dr A obtains a medically appropriate history from the parents. An examination is accomplished. The patient has multiple allergies to medications, and extensive research with the pharmacist is required to determine appropriate antibiotics for treatment. Dr A spends 35 total minutes seeing the patient and researching antibiotics, discussing options with the pharmacist, and documenting the encounter. Using time as the basis for code selection, which E/M code(s) should be reported for this case study?

Case Study 9

Dr F sees a 56-year-old established patient with stable exertional angina who complains of new-onset calf pain while walking. A history including other episodes of chest pain or difficulty breathing and a physical examination including neurologic status and gait evaluation are performed. Options to diagnose the condition and potential therapy are explained to the patient. Dr F spends 30 total minutes on the day of the encounter with the patient, including ordering an ankle-brachial index test and documenting the encounter. Using time as the basis for code selection, which E/M code(s) should be reported for this case study?

Case Study 10

A 50-year-old female with dyspepsia and nausea is seen by Dr S as a new patient. A history is obtained, and a relevant exam is performed. Diagnostic tests are arranged, and follow-up with the patient is scheduled after lengthy discussion about timing of meals, medications, and lifestyle modification. Dr S spends a total of 38 minutes on the day of the encounter. Using time as the basis for code selection, which E/M code(s) should be reported for this case study?

SECTION 4

E/M 2021: Prolonged Services and Code-Level Selection Changes

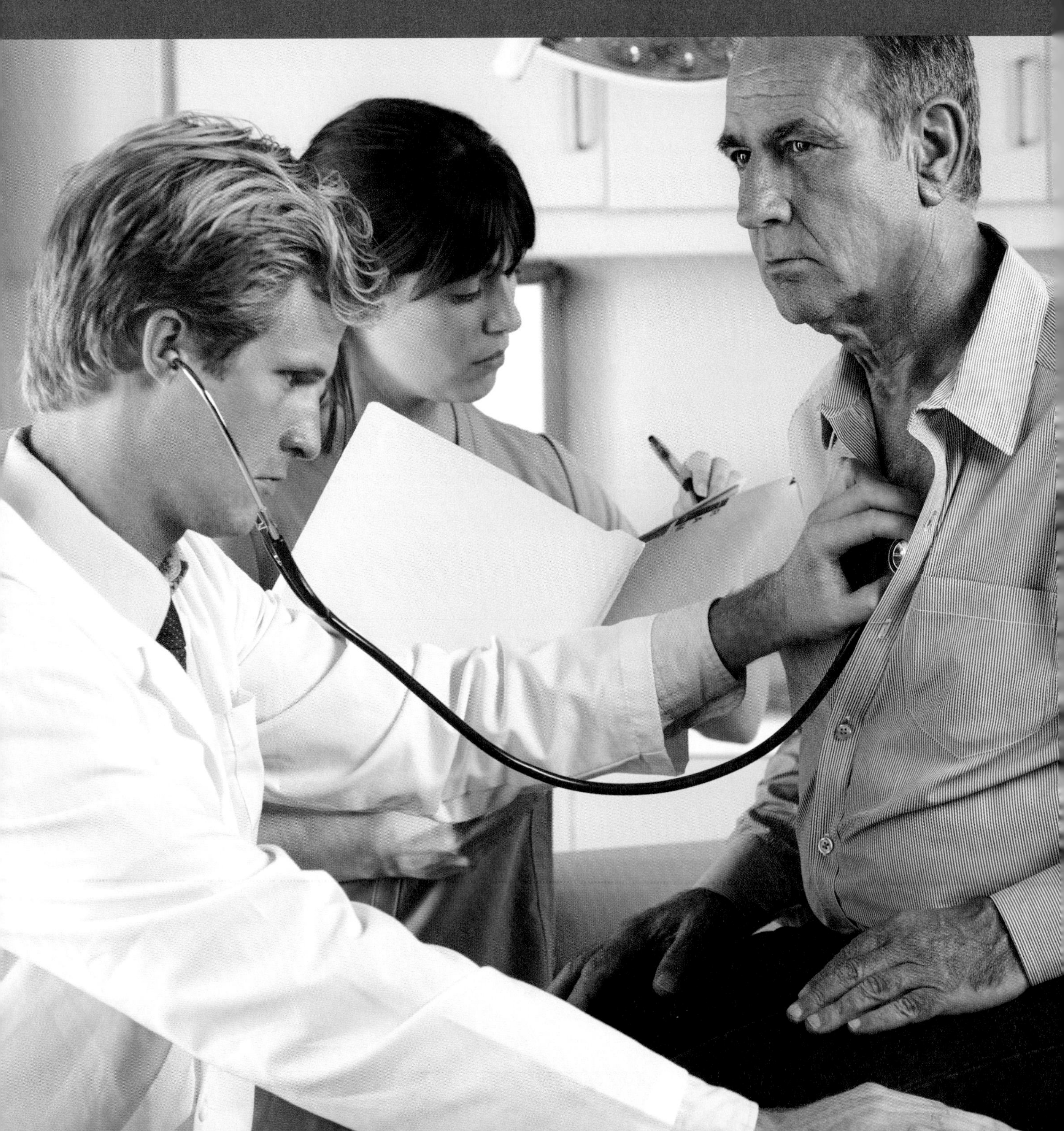

The creation of a new prolonged services code, combined with changes to the descriptors of the evaluation and management (E/M) office or other outpatient visit codes, necessitated revisions in many of the other prolonged services guidelines, code descriptors, and parentheticals. This chapter reviews and highlights these changes, including updates for reporting time of physicians, other qualified health care professionals (QHPs), and clinical staff. In addition, this chapter also analyzes the effects of each revision on other codes, both within prolonged services and across other E/M code groups. It is absolutely essential to refer to the official E/M guidelines and E/M services in Section 5 of this book and to read the revised guidelines in full to ensure complete understanding of all the changes.

The objectives of this section are as follows:

- Gain in-depth knowledge of the new shorter prolonged services code and know when to use it
- Understand the range of prolonged services codes and how they are affected by the 2021 changes
- Use the quick-reference reporting table to pair the prolonged services code(s) with their associated E/M code(s)

CHAPTER 4

Prolonged Services

Overview

The need to identify situations in which the service provided in a category or subcategory of E/M goes beyond what is usually required is not a new concept. The E/M changes in 1992 introduced a modifier to identify prolonged services specifically to be used with E/M services codes. Following that change, five-digit Current Procedural Terminology (CPT®) codes to replace the modifier were established in 1994. Since then, revisions to the prolonged services codes have provided further clarification and delineation of their uses with other E/M codes.

To facilitate proper application of the prolonged services codes, the code descriptors and/or their guidelines or parenthetical notes include the following key information:

- Whether the prolonged service involves direct patient contact
- The service setting for the primary E/M service (eg, inpatient, outpatient, observation)
- The amount of time of the prolonged service
- The date of the additional service relative to the primary E/M service
- The CPT E/M codes to which the prolonged services codes apply

As discussed in Chapters 2 and 3, the most significant E/M changes for 2021 pertain to the office and other outpatient codes 99202-99215 and the use of either time or medical decision making (MDM) to select the appropriate level for code selection. In the process of making changes to those E/M office and other outpatient codes, the CPT Editorial Panel also identified the need for a shorter-duration prolonged service(s) code, with an appropriate shorter time interval (ie, 15 minutes) (as opposed to the time in the existing codes before 2021, which describe intervals of 1 hour and longer) to capture the additional time and work commonly required for these encounters.

New Shorter Prolonged Service(s) Code

The new prolonged office or other outpatient E/M service(s) code (99417) and its descriptor and all related parenthetical notes are provided as follows.

▶Prolonged Service With or Without Direct Patient Contact on the Date of an Office or Other Outpatient Service◀

#★+●99417 Prolonged office or other outpatient evaluation and management service(s) beyond the minimum required time of the primary procedure which has been selected using total time, requiring total time with or without direct patient contact beyond the usual service, on the date of the primary service, each 15 minutes of total time (List separately in addition to codes 99205, 99215 for office or other outpatient **Evaluation and Management** services)

▶(Use 99417 in conjunction with 99205, 99215)◀

▶(Do not report 99417 on the same date of service as 99354, 99355, 99358, 99359, 99415, 99416)◀

▶(Do not report 99417 for any time unit less than 15 minutes)◀

Some of the key instructions for using code 99417 include the following:

- Code 99417 should be reported for prolonged office or other outpatient services only when time is used as the basis for code selection. This code may not be used when MDM is used as the basis for code selection.
- Code 99417 may be used only with the highest-level office or other outpatient services (ie, 99205 [new patient] or 99215 [established patient]), and only when the time required to report those services has been exceeded by 15 minutes.
- Prolonged services of less than 15 minutes of total time on the date of the office or other outpatient service (99205 or 99215) may not be reported.
- Time spent performing services reported separately from the E/M service may not be counted toward the time to report codes 99205 and 99215 or any prolonged services codes.

Table 1 provides guidance on the use of new code 99417 (prolonged office or other outpatient E/M service[s]) with code 99205 (new patient). Remember that the time applied toward the new prolonged service(s) code 99417 does not begin until the requirements for reporting the base E/M visit code have been met. In the case of a new patient encounter (99205), 60 minutes of time are required to report the service. Do not report code 99417 until at least 15 minutes of time have been accumulated beyond the required 60 minutes (ie, 75 minutes) on the date of the encounter.

ADVICE/ALERT NOTE

Remember that the time applied toward the new prolonged service(s) code 99417 does not begin until the requirements for reporting the base E/M visit code have been met. For a new patient encounter (99205), 60 minutes of time are required to report the service.

CODING TIP Do not report code 99417 until at least 15 minutes of time has been accumulated beyond the required 60 minutes (ie, 75 minutes) on the date of the encounter.

Prolonged Services

TABLE 1 Use of Code 99417 With Code 99205

▶Total Duration of New Patient Office or Other Outpatient Services (use with 99205)	Code(s)
less than 75 minutes	Not reported separately
75-89 minutes	99205 X 1 and 99417 X 1
90-104 minutes	99205 X 1 and 99417 X 2
105 minutes or more	99205 X 1 and 99417 X 3 or more for each additional 15 minutes

CODING TIP For an established patient encounter (99215), 40 minutes of time are required to report the service. Do not report code 99417 until at least 15 minutes of time has been accumulated beyond the required 40 minutes (ie, 55 minutes) on the date of the encounter.

Table 2 provides reporting guidance for the new shorter prolonged service(s) code 99417 with code 99215 (established patient).

TABLE 2 Use of Code 99417 With Code 99215

Total Duration of Established Patient Office or Other Outpatient Services (use with 99215)	Code(s)
less than 55 minutes	Not reported separately
55-69 minutes	99215 X 1 and 99417 X 1
70-84 minutes	99215 X 1 and 99417 X 2
85 minutes or more	99215 X 1 and 99417 X 3 or more for each additional 15 minutes◀

ADVICE/ALERT NOTE

For shorter time periods for prolonged services for both new and established patients, do not use time for code selection.

Table 3 provides a summary of how to report the new shorter prolonged service(s) code with the E/M office or other outpatient codes for 2021 when time is the basis for code selection. Note that for the shorter time periods for both new and established patients, time is not used for code selection.

TABLE 3 Summary of Prolonged Services Reporting Based on Time

Type of Patient	Time (Minutes)						
New Patient	1-14	15-29	30-44	45-59	60-74	75-89	90-104
	Do not use time (report 99202 by MDM)	99202	99203	99204	99205 (reporting requirement met at 60 minutes)	99205 + 99417	99205 + 99417 ×2
Established Patient	1-9	10-19	20-29	30-39	40-54	55-69	70-84
	Do not use time (report 99212 by MDM)	99212	99213	99214	99215 (reporting requirement met at 40 min)	99215 + 99417	99215 + 99417 ×2

Related Prolonged Services Reporting: Physicians and Other Qualified Health Care Professionals

Prolonged services codes can be reported in a variety of settings and applications. For example, they may be reported with E/M codes for certain inpatient services, and on days other than the date of the primary service. While only one new, shorter prolonged service(s) code has been created for 2021, that addition, as well as revisions of the base E/M codes it is used with, has led to changes in many of the other existing prolonged services codes. For the other existing prolonged services codes, parenthetical instructions have been added to specify whether those codes may be reported with the new E/M office or other outpatient codes; additional revisions are specific to the code being described.

A list of the revised descriptors and parenthetical notes for CPT 2021 covering prolonged services codes 99354-99359 that may be reported by physicians and/or other QHPs is provided below.

▶Prolonged Service With Direct Patient Contact (Except with Office or Other Outpatient Services)◀

★+▲99354 Prolonged service(s) in the outpatient setting requiring direct patient contact beyond the time of the usual service; first hour (List separately in addition to code for outpatient **Evaluation and Management** or psychotherapy service, except with office or other outpatient services [99202, 99203, 99204, 99205, 99212, 99213, 99214, 99215])

▶(Use 99354 in conjunction with 90837, 90847, 99241-99245, 99324-99337, 99341-99350, 99483)◀

▶(Do not report 99354 in conjunction with 99202, 99203, 99204, 99205, 99212, 99213, 99214, 99215, 99415, 99416, 99417)◀

★+▲99355 each additional 30 minutes (List separately in addition to code for prolonged service)

(Use 99355 in conjunction with 99354)

▶(Do not report 99355 in conjunction with 99202, 99203, 99204, 99205, 99212, 99213, 99214, 99215, 99415, 99416, 99417)◀

+▲99356 Prolonged service in the inpatient or observation setting, requiring unit/floor time beyond the usual service; first hour (List separately in addition to code for inpatient or observation **Evaluation and Management** service)

▶(Use 99356 in conjunction with 90837, 90847, 99218-99220, 99221-99223, 99224-99226, 99231-99233, 99234-99236, 99251-99255, 99304-99310)◀

+99357 each additional 30 minutes (List separately in addition to code for prolonged service)

(Use 99357 in conjunction with 99356)

(continued)

ADVICE/ALERT NOTE

Prolonged services codes can be reported in a variety of settings and applications. For example, they may be reported with E/M codes for certain inpatient services, and on days other than the date of the primary service.

CODING TIP Code 99354 may be reported with the following services:

- Psychotherapy (90837, 90847)
- Office consultation (99241-99245)
- Domiciliary or rest home visit (99324-99337)
- Home visit evaluation and management (99341-99350)
- Evaluation and care plans for symptoms of cognitive impairment (99483)

 **ADVICE/ALERT NOTE**

Prolonged services without direct patient contact (99358, 99359) may be reported with E/M office or other outpatient codes (99202-99215) *only* when the prolonged services occur on a date other than the primary office E/M service.

Prolonged Service Without Direct Patient Contact

99358 **Prolonged evaluation and management service** before and/or after direct patient care; first hour

+99359 each additional 30 minutes (List separately in addition to code for prolonged service)

(Use 99359 in conjunction with 99358)

►(Do not report 99358, 99359 on the same date of service as 99202, 99203, 99204, 99205, 99212, 99213, 99214, 99215, 99417)◄

CPT codes 99354 and 99355 are used to report the total duration of *face-to-face* time in the outpatient setting spent by a physician or other QHP on a given date providing prolonged service even if the time spent by the physician or other QHP on that date is not continuous. These codes may be reported in addition to the appropriate outpatient E/M, psychotherapy, domiciliary or rest home, and/or home care services, as well as services for cognitive assessment and care plans. *Note that the parentheticals added for these codes specifically exclude reporting with codes 99202-99205 or 99212-99215 or when any related prolonged services code is used.*

Codes 99356 and 99357 are used to report the total duration of prolonged services provided to a patient by a physician or other QHP at the bedside and on the patient's floor or unit on a given date in an inpatient facility or observation setting (eg, hospital or nursing facility), even if the time spent by the physician or other QHP on that date is not continuous. The revision of these codes involved modifications to clarify their use specifically with codes for inpatient or observation E/M services.

ADVICE/ALERT NOTE

The prolonged non-face-to-face time must relate to face-to-face patient care that has occurred or will occur and must relate to ongoing patient management.

Codes 99358 and 99359 are used when a prolonged service is provided without direct patient contact, ie, neither face-to-face time in the outpatient, inpatient, or observation setting, nor additional unit or floor time in a facility or observation setting. These codes may be reported with E/M office or other outpatient codes (99202-99215) *only* when the prolonged services occur on a date other than the primary E/M office service. Codes 99358 and 99359 may be reported on the same date as an E/M service, *except* for office or other outpatient services (99202-99205, 99212-99215). The prolonged service may be reported on a different date than the primary service to which it is related, *including* office or other outpatient services (99202-99205, 99212-99215). For example, extensive record review may relate to a previous E/M service performed on an earlier date or an upcoming E/M service on a future date.

Codes 99358 and 99359 are used to report the total duration of non-face-to-face time spent by the reporting physician or other QHP providing prolonged service on a given date, even if the time spent by the physician or other QHP on that date is not continuous. Code 99358 is used to report the first hour of prolonged service on a given date regardless of the place of service and may only be reported once per date.

Related Prolonged Services Reporting: Clinical Staff

The prolonged services performed by clinical staff may be reported under certain conditions. This includes the requirement for physician or other QHP supervision in the office setting. The following list shows the revised descriptors and parenthetical notes for codes 99415-99416 in CPT 2021 for reporting prolonged clinical staff time.

#+▲99415 Prolonged clinical staff service (the service beyond the highest time in the range of total time of the service) during an evaluation and management service in the office or outpatient setting, direct patient contact with physician supervision; first hour (List separately in addition to code for outpatient **Evaluation and Management** service)

▶(Use 99415 in conjunction with 99202, 99203, 99204, 99205, 99212, 99213, 99214, 99215)◀

▶(Do not report 99415 in conjunction with 99354, 99355, 99417)◀

#+▲99416 each additional 30 minutes (List separately in addition to code for prolonged service)

(Use 99416 in conjunction with 99415)

▶(Do not report 99416 in conjunction with 99354, 99355, 99417)◀

Codes 99415 and 99416 are designed specifically for use in the office setting, and therefore, they are limited for use with the E/M office or other outpatient codes. Revisions in the code descriptor reflect a change in the time reference of the primary E/M service codes, from typical time to total time. Table 4 illustrates the correct reporting of prolonged services provided by clinical staff with physician or other QHP supervision in the office setting beyond the first 30 minutes of clinical staff time.

TABLE 4 Use of Codes 99415 and 99416: Prolonged Services by Clinical Staff

Total Duration of Prolonged Services	Code(s)
less than 30 minutes	Not reported separately
30-74 minutes (30 minutes - 1 hr. 14 min.)	99415 X 1
75-104 minutes (1 hr. 15 min. - 1 hr. 44 min.)	99415 X 1 AND 99416 X 1
105 minutes or more (1 hr. 45 min. or more)	99415 X 1 AND 99416 X 2 or more for each additional 30 minutes.◀

CODING TIP The new prolonged service code 99417 may only be reported with either code 99205 or 99215, and it includes total physician and/or QHP face-to-face and non-face-to-face E/M services on the date of the encounter.

Accordingly, neither the face-to-face prolonged services codes (99354, 99355) nor the non-face-to-face codes (99358, 99359) may be reported on the same date as the office or other outpatient services (99202-99205, 99212-99215). Codes 99358 and 99359 may continue to be reported on a date *other than* the date of the encounter.

ADVICE/ALERT NOTE

Revisions in the code descriptors of 99415 and 99416 reflect a change in the time reference of the primary E/M service codes, ie, from typical time to total time.

 **ADVICE/ALERT NOTE**

When using prolonged services codes, remember that for a time-based add-on code to be used or reported, the primary E/M service code must have a typical or specified time published in the CPT code set; this is usually listed in the code description. A specified time is needed in order to distinguish between the time spent on the primary service and the time allotted to the prolonged service. The appropriate time should be documented in the medical record when it is used as the basis for code selection.

CODING TIP Prolonged services may not be reported with codes 99384-99397 (preventive services) or codes 99281-99285 (emergency department) because these codes have no specified time as part of the code description.

ADVICE/ALERT NOTE

The code selection criteria related to time have not been altered for other E/M services. Review and refer to the appropriate CPT codes and descriptors for the correct typical time.

When using prolonged services codes, remember that for a time-based add-on code to be used or reported, the primary E/M service code must have a typical or specified time published in the CPT code set; this is usually listed in the code description. A specified time is needed in order to distinguish between the time spent on the primary service and the time allotted to the prolonged services code.

Prolonged services may not be reported with preventive services codes 99384-99397 or emergency department codes 99281-99285 because these codes have no specified time as part of the code description.

Prolonged Services Reporting Across E/M Code Groups

The E/M guidelines for reporting time are in the Evaluation and Management (E/M) Services Guidelines section of the *CPT 2021* codebook. This section includes the revised guidelines for E/M codes 99202-99205 and 99211-99215.

When prolonged services are provided, the appropriate prolonged services code must be selected and reported in addition to the primary E/M service code. A summary of prolonged services codes and the associated E/M service code groups is included in Section 5 of this book and is also provided in Table 5.

TABLE 5 ►Comparison of Prolonged Services Codes (99354, 99355, 99356, 99357, 99358, 99359, 99417) Table◄

►Code	Patient Contact	Minimum Reportable Prolonged Services Time (Single Date of Service)	Use In Conjunction With	*Do Not Report With	Other Prolonged Service(s) Reportable On Same Date Of Service
+99354	Face-to-Face Only	30 minutes (Beyond listed typical time)	90837, 90847, 99241-99245, 99324-99337, 99341-99350, 99483	99202-99205, 99212-99215, 99415, 99416, 99417	99358, 99359
+99355	Face-to-Face Only	Each additional 15 minutes (Beyond 99354)	99354	99202-99205, 99212-99215, 99415, 99416, 99417	99358, 99359
+99356	Face-to-Face and Unit/Floor Time	30 minutes (Beyond listed typical time)	90837, 90847, 99218-99220, 99221-99223, 99224-99226, 99231-99233, 99234-99236, 99251-99255, 99304-99310		99358, 99359
+99357	Face-to-Face and Unit/Floor Time	Each additional 15 minutes (Beyond 99356)	99356		99358, 99359
99358	Non-Face-to-Face Only	30 minutes	Must relate to a service where face-to-face care has or will occur. This is not an add-on code and is not used in conjunction with a base code.	99202-99205, 99212-99215, 99417 On same date of service	99354, 99356
+99359	Non-Face-to-Face Only	Each additional 15 minutes (Beyond 99358)	99358	99202-99205, 99212-99215, 99417 On same date of service	99354, 99356
+99417	Face-to-Face and/or Non-Face-to-Face	Reported with 99205: 75 minutes or more Reported with 99215: 55 minutes or more ***(Total time on the date of encounter)***	99205, 99215	99354, 99355, 99358, 99359, 99415, 99416	N/A

*Do not count the time of any separately reported service as prolonged services time
99355 is for prolonged services time beyond 99354 and may be reported in multiple units
99357 is for prolonged services time beyond 99356 and may be reported in multiple units
99359 is for prolonged services time beyond 99358 and may be reported in multiple units
99417 is for prolonged services time beyond 99205 or 99215 and may be reported in multiple units of at least 15 minutes◄

Evaluate Your Understanding

The following questions and case studies are critical checkpoints that are meant to let you apply your critical thinking and evaluate your understanding of the content covered in the chapter. The answers for the end-of-chapter exercises are available at amaproductupdates.org.

A Multiple Choice Questions

Select the correct or most appropriate answer(s) to the following questions.

1. Which of the following codes describes a prolonged service in the inpatient or observation setting, requiring unit/floor time beyond the usual service; first hour (List separately in addition to code for inpatient or observation **Evaluation and Management** service)?
   a. 99355
   b. 99416
   c. 99417
   d. 99356

2. Which of the following is the code descriptor for code 99358?
   a. **Prolonged evaluation and management service** before and/or after direct patient care; first hour
   b. **Office or other outpatient visit** for the evaluation and management of an established patient, which requires a medically appropriate history and/or examination and high level of medical decision making
   c. Prolonged clinical staff service (the service beyond the highest time in the range of total time of the service) during an evaluation and management service in the office or outpatient setting, direct patient contact with physician supervision; first hour (List separately in addition to code for outpatient **Evaluation and Management** service)
   d. None of the above

3. Which code represents prolonged service(s) in the outpatient setting requiring direct patient contact beyond the time of the usual service; first hour (List separately in addition to code for outpatient Evaluation and Management or psychotherapy service, except with office or other outpatient services [99202, 99203, 99204, 99205, 99212, 99213, 99214, 99215])?
   a. 99359
   b. 99354
   c. 99355
   d. 99357

4. Which code represents prolonged service(s) in the outpatient setting requiring direct patient contact beyond the time of the usual service; each additional 30 minutes (List separately in addition to code for prolonged service)?
   a. 99416
   b. 99417
   c. 99355
   d. 99356

5. Which code represents prolonged office or other outpatient evaluation and management service(s) beyond the minimum required time of the primary procedure which has been selected using total time, requiring total time with or without direct patient contact beyond the usual service, on the date of the primary service, each 15 minutes of total time (List separately in addition to codes 99205, 99215 for office or other outpatient Evaluation and Management services)?
   a. 99357
   b. 99417
   c. 99355
   d. 99415

Prolonged Services

6. Which code represents prolonged evaluation and management service before and/or after direct patient care; each additional 30 minutes (List separately in addition to code for prolonged service)?
   a. 99356
   b. 99357
   c. 99358
   d. 99359

7. Which code represents prolonged clinical staff service (the service beyond the highest time in the range of total time of the service) during an evaluation and management service in the office or outpatient setting, direct patient contact with physician supervision; first hour (List separately in addition to code for outpatient Evaluation and Management service)?
   a. 99354
   b. 99355
   c. 99416
   d. 99415

8. Which code represents prolonged service in the inpatient or observation setting, requiring unit/floor time beyond the usual service; each additional 30 minutes (List separately in addition to code for prolonged service)?
   a. 99357
   b. 99358
   c. 99354
   d. 99416

9. Which code represents prolonged clinical staff service (the service beyond the highest time in the range of total time of the service) during an evaluation and management service in the office or outpatient setting, direct patient contact with physician supervision; each additional 30 minutes (List separately in addition to code for prolonged service)?
   a. 99416
   b. 99417
   c. 99356
   d. 99358

B True/False Questions

Answer true (T) or false (F) to the following statements.

1. _____ The new prolonged services code 99417 is structured in 15-minute increments.

2. _____ Prolonged services code 99417 may be reported when either medical decision making or time is used to select the primary level of service.

3. _____ Code 99417 may only be reported with codes 99205 and 99215.

4. _____ Prolonged services codes 99354 and 99355 are reported for total face-to-face time by a physician or other qualified health care professional (QHP) on a given date of service even if the time spent is not continuous.

5. _____ Prolonged services codes 99356 and 99357 are reported for total duration of time spent by a physician or other QHP at the bedside and on the patient's floor or unit in the hospital or nursing facility on a given date only if the time spent is continuous.

6. _____ Prolonged services codes 99358 and 99359 are reported for services that involve neither face-to-face time in the outpatient, inpatient, or observation setting nor additional unit/floor time in the hospital or nursing facility setting.

7. _____ For an established patient encounter (99215), 40 minutes of time are required to report the service. Prolonged services code 99417 may be reported when the encounter reaches 55 minutes of service time.

8. _____ Codes 99358 and 99359 may be reported on a different date than the primary service to which it is related for codes other than 99202-99215.

9. _____ For codes 99358 and 99359, extensive record review may not be a criterion for reporting prolonged services that relate to an E/M service performed on an earlier date.

10. _____ For a new patient encounter (99205), 60 minutes of time are required to report the service. Prolonged services code 99417 may be reported when the encounter reaches 75 minutes of service time.

11. _____ Code 99358 is used to report the first hour of prolonged services on a given date regardless of the place of service.

12. _____ Neither the face-to-face prolonged services codes (99354 and 99355) nor the non-face-to-face codes (99358 and 99359) may be reported on the same date as the office or other outpatient services (99202-99205, 99212-99215).

C Fill in the Blank

Fill in the blank in the following statements with the most correct response.

1. Prolonged services code 99417 may be reported for services _______________ direct patient contact on the date of the encounter.
2. Time spent performing separately reported services other than the E/M service _______________ (will/will not) be counted toward the time to report code 99205, code 99215, and prolonged services time.
3. In order to report code 99417 with code 99205, _______________ minutes must have been reached.
4. Prolonged services codes 99358 and 99359 may be reported on a different _______________ than the primary service to which the code is related.
5. Prolonged services codes 99415 and 99416 are reported when an E/M service provided in the office or outpatient setting involves prolonged face-to-face time by _______________ beyond the highest total time of the E/M service, as stated in the ranges of time in the code descriptions.
6. When reporting codes 99415 and 99416, the physician must be present to provide direct _______________ of the clinical staff.
7. Prolonged services codes 99354 and 99355 may not be reported in conjunction with codes _______________.
8. Code 99356, *Prolonged service in the inpatient or observation setting, requiring unit/floor time beyond the usual service*, is reported for the _______________ of time.
9. Codes 99356 and 99357 are reported for prolonged services performed in the _______________.
10. In order to report code 99417 with code 99215, _______________ minutes must have been reached.
11. In order to use or report time-based add-on codes, the primary E/M service code must have a _______________ listed in the code's description.
12. Prolonged face-to-face clinical staff services (codes 99415, 99416) of less than _______________ minutes are not reported separately.

Prolonged Services

D Internet-based Exercises 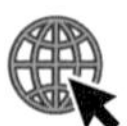

1. For additional information regarding 2021 E/M prolonged services, see https://codingintel.com/are-changes-coming-for-prolonged-services/#:~:text=The%20AMA%20has%20developed%20a,and%20CMS%20documents%20as%2099XXX.
2. For more useful advice for 2021 E/M prolonged services, visit https://www.mdedge.com/gihepnews/article/217817/practice-management/prepare-major-changes-e/m-coding-starting-2021.
3. For additional information about the changes in the 2021 E/M prolonged services, see https://quizlet.com/72646384/cpt-em-prolonged-services-flash-cards/.
4. For the basics of prolonged services before the changes for E/M 2021, visit https://www.aapc.com/blog/38738-hard-facts-of-coding-prolonged-services/.
5. For helpful information, chart, and tables that show how to select prolonged services codes, check out https://practice.asco.org/sites/default/files/drupalfiles/2020-06/NewProlongedEM%20FINAL.pdf.

E Short Answer Questions

Answer the following questions with the most correct response.

1. Can we report the new prolonged services code 99417 for a new patient visit that required 72 minutes of total time?
2. Would it be appropriate to report the new prolonged services code 99417 for an established patient visit that required 65 minutes of total time?
3. Is the new prolonged services code 99417 intended to be used with other prolonged services codes such as 99354 or 99355?
4. May the new prolonged services code 99417 be used with E/M emergency department service codes (99281-99285)?
5. Is there a coding mechanism available to report prolonged services that are performed by clinical staff under physician supervision? For example, a patient required extended direct patient contact totaling 60 minutes provided by a nurse.
6. What code(s) may be reported for prolonged services that are neither face-to-face time in the outpatient, inpatient, or observation setting nor additional unit/floor time in a facility or observation setting and that are provided on a different date than the primary service to which they are related?
7. What codes exist to report a total of 60 minutes of prolonged services by a physician or other qualified health care professional (QHP) at the bedside or on the patient's floor or unit, in a facility inpatient or observation setting (eg, hospital or nursing facility) on a given date?
8. A physician spent an additional 35 minutes of face-to-face time beyond 75 minutes with a patient in an assisted living facility, providing prolonged services. In addition to the appropriate E/M code (eg, 99328), are there any codes that can be reported for this situation?
9. Is it appropriate to report prolonged services codes for an office visit when additional time is spent by the physician to perform a separate procedure, such as debriding and dressing a simple wound (eg, 12001-12021), or preparing and delivering injections or infusions (90760-90779)?
10. Would it be appropriate to count prolonged services time from multiple dates to arrive at a total time for reporting prolonged services codes 99354-99357?

Prolonged Services

F Case Studies

Although each of the following scenarios may involve service(s) or procedure(s) besides E/M, code only the E/M services. Use the *CPT 2021* codebook to determine the correct code(s) to report the E/M service(s) associated with each of the following procedure(s) or service(s).

Case Study 1

A hospitalized patient experiences a change in condition. The patient was seen previously in the day, and 25 minutes were spent at the hospital unit performing services reported with code 99232. The physician returns to the unit and spends 55 minutes assessing the patient and discussing the matter with the patient and family, who are also in attendance. Which E/M code(s) should be reported for this case study?

Case Study 2

A 40-year-old female with acute rheumatoid arthritis and deteriorating function is seen by her physician for a follow-up visit in the office. The physician spends a total of 55 minutes reviewing external notes and talking with the patient and her family about her condition and additional treatment options along with their risks and benefits. The patient is quite concerned about her functional decline, and referrals for occupational and physical therapy are generated. Which E/M code(s) should be reported for this case study?

Case Study 3

During an office visit for an established patient, the physician spends 45 minutes counseling and educating the patient and family on post-stroke care for the patient, who has suffered a debilitating stroke. Because the physician lacks some details about the stroke etiology and consults performed during inpatient treatment, records are requested. Nine days after the visit, the physician spends an hour on a single date extensively reviewing the patient's records obtained after the previous visit. Which E/M code(s) should be reported for this case study?

Case Study 4

An established patient with anxiety and depression was seen for administration of intranasal esketamine. The physician documented an appropriate history and relevant examination and counseled the patient regarding this treatment option for 20 minutes. Medication was given in the office setting following the assessment; after it was given, clinical staff observed the patient to look for changes in physiological response or side effects. The physician supervised the clinical staff during this time. The total time for the monitoring was 60 minutes of clinical staff time spent face to face with the patient and not performing any other reportable services. Which E/M code(s) should be reported for this case study?

Case Study 5

A 69-year-old male with severe chronic obstructive pulmonary disease, congestive heart failure, and hypertension presented to the office for a new patient visit. Dr M took an extensive history due to the patient's multiple medical issues including a review of prior treatment, tests, and other details from the patient's old records. A physical examination was performed, and there was a lengthy discussion with the patient about multisystem illness severity and the prognosis without adequate treatment and follow-up. Counseling including smoking, diet, and medication compliance was performed. Dr M completed medical record documentation with plans to refer the patient to a pulmonary medicine and cardiology subspecialist after test results are received. The total time spent with the patient was 92 minutes. Which E/M code(s) should be reported for this case study?

Case Study 6

A 63-year-old established patient with type 2 diabetes mellitus, congestive heart failure, hyperlipidemia, and chronic anxiety presented to Dr P's office with complaints of blurred vision, frequent urination, high blood sugars, and left leg pain and swelling. Dr P reviewed the medical history form completed by the patient and vital signs obtained by clinical staff. A relevant interval history was obtained, including response to treatment at last visit, and an appropriate physical examination was performed. A new treatment plan was developed. Dr P wrote multiple prescriptions and arranged for laboratory work to be performed. Dr P spent extensive time with the patient discussing the details of each condition, the options for additional management, and the associated risks. Documentation was entered into the electronic medical record. Dr P sent updated correspondence to the patient's neurologist and cardiologist and added a reminder to check the patient's test results. The total time spent on the encounter was 74 minutes. Which E/M code(s) should be reported for this case study?

Case Study 7

A 65-year-old new patient with multiple complicated medical problems was brought to Dr K's office by her daughter. The physician reviewed the medical history form completed by the patient and vital signs obtained by the medical assistant. The patient's history was verified with some independent history obtained from the daughter when the patient was unable to recall details of her previous care, and an appropriate examination was performed. A tentative treatment plan was developed based on review of available notes, with the expectation that it would be revised, if necessary, pending review of outside records that were requested and the results of the diagnostic tests and laboratory work that were ordered during this encounter. A discussion was held with the patient and her daughter regarding the potential management options, risks related both to the condition and to the treatment choices, and reassessment of current medications the patient is taking. The encounter was appropriately documented in the medical record. The medical decision making was moderate, and the total time spent on this encounter was 50 minutes. Several weeks after the visit, the physician spent 45 minutes on a single day reviewing detailed medical records transferred from the patient's previous physicians, completing a revised treatment plan, and talking with the daughter. Which E/M code(s) should be reported for this case study?

Case Study 8

A 52-year-old female established patient presents to the office with gastroenteritis and persistent vomiting. She also shows signs and symptoms of clinical dehydration. Dr A spends 15 minutes assessing the patient and formulating a treatment plan. The decision is made to begin oral rehydration in the office. The LPN performs prolonged monitoring and observation for 80 minutes under the physician's supervision with intermittent evaluation of the patient by Dr A. Which E/M code(s) should be reported for this case study?

Case Study 9

A 34-year-old primigravida is seen in the hospital unit with severe preeclampsia. The physician supervises management of the preeclampsia with intravenous magnesium initiation and maintenance, labor augmentation with oxytocin, and close maternal-fetal monitoring. The physician provides continuous bedside care until the patient is stable and then provides intermittent care for the next 90 minutes until the delivery. Care involves patient evaluation, monitoring and interpretation of laboratory results, and adjustment of therapy as needed. Which E/M code(s) should be reported for this case study?

Case Study 10

A 53-year-old female established patient presents to the office complaining of joint pain and fatigue, which have increased in frequency over the past month, with her daughter who serves as her interpreter because she has a limited ability to speak and understand English. She is well and otherwise stable, being managed for diabetes mellitus type 2 and asthma; the patient underwent a total thyroidectomy approximately 2 years ago. The family practice physician reviews the patient's latest thyroid-stimulating hormone (TSH), metabolic panel, pulmonary function tests results, and vital signs obtained by a medical assistant. An elevated blood pressure reading of 145/93 is noted, which the patient attributes to a stressful drive to the physician's office.

The physician performs a medically appropriate physical examination to assess the joint pain and fatigue and creates and discusses with the patient a treatment plan to address both problems. Following the assessment, the physician again measures the patient's blood pressure, allowing time for the effects of the drive to dissipate during the visit; the second reading is 145/95. Upon further discussion, the patient notes that she had received similar readings 2 and 3 weeks ago when attempting to donate blood. The physician conducts an additional evaluation, makes a diagnosis of stage 2 hypertension, and begins a dual medication regimen to address the patient's hypertension, taking the patient's current drug regimen into account. The patient is also counseled on needed lifestyle changes. The patient encounter takes a total of 42 minutes, given the additional problem identified during the visit and the need for an interpreter. Later in the day, the physician spends 5 minutes discussing the patient's joint-pain symptoms with a rheumatologist that the physician frequently works with, an additional 6 minutes on documentation and revision of the treatment plan, including ordering a sleep study to further evaluate for potential sleep apnea, and 4 minutes on a telephone call with the patient's daughter to inform her of her mother's test results, and the need to arrange for the patient to undergo the sleep study. Which E/M code(s) should be reported for this case study?

SECTION 5

E/M Guidelines and Codes

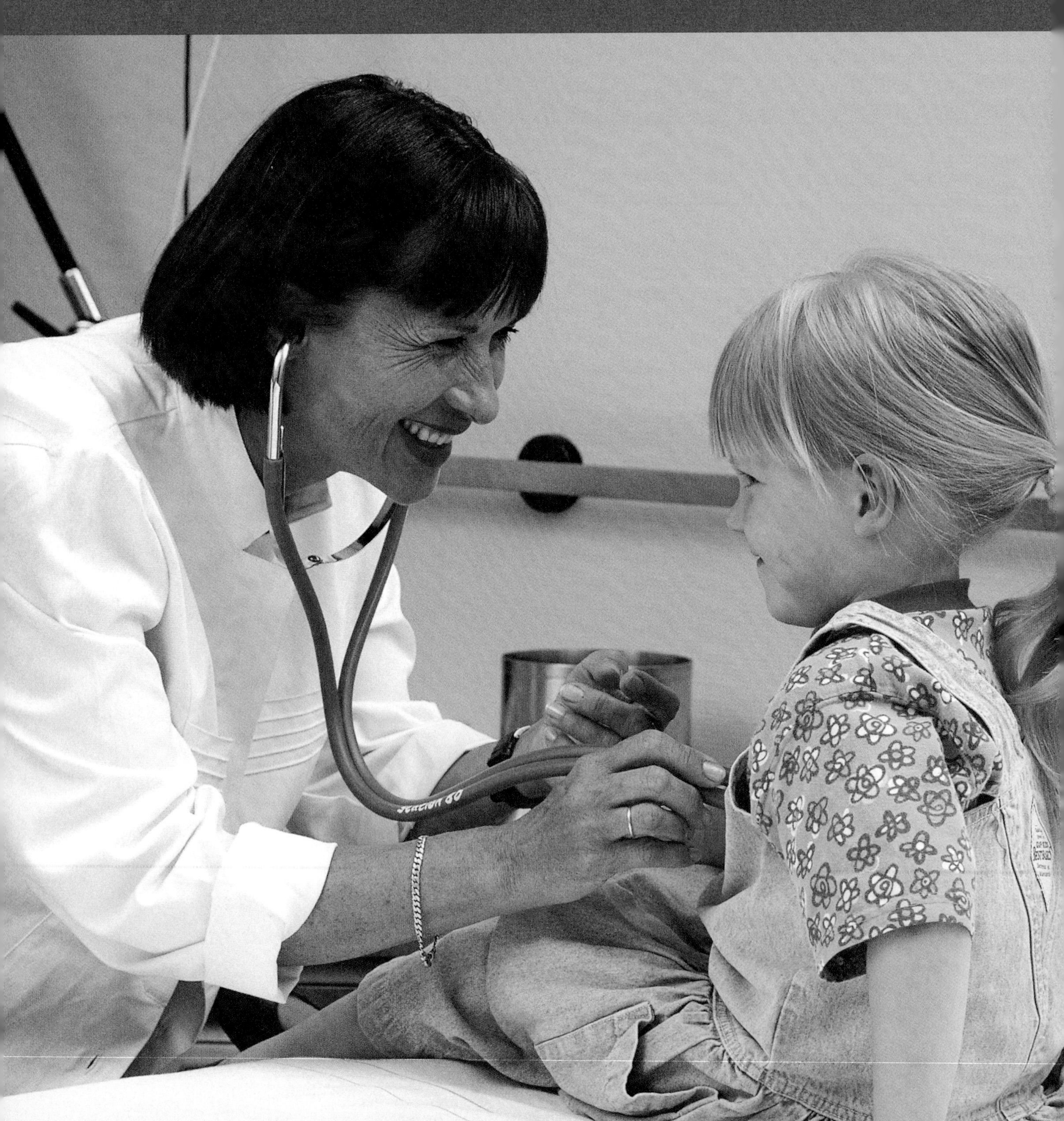

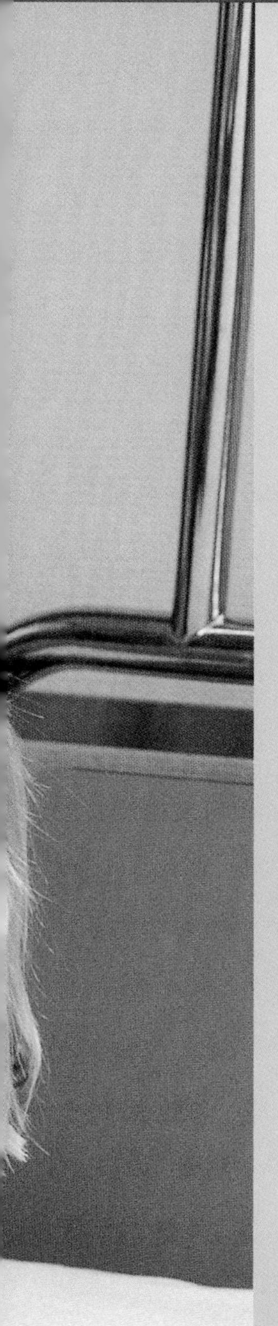

This section consists of two chapters and is intended to provide reference copies of the official evaluation and management (E/M) materials from the *Current Procedural Terminology (CPT®) 2021 Professional (CPT 2021)* codebook in an effort to make this book a comprehensive resource for the revised E/M code set.

The objectives of this section are as follows:

- Reference the full set of official E/M 2021 guidelines, as published in the *CPT 2021* codebook
- Ensure quick access to the entire E/M section's codes

CHAPTER 5

Evaluation and Management (E/M) Services Guidelines

In addition to the information presented in the Introduction [of the *CPT 2021* codebook], several other items unique to this section are defined or identified here.

▸E/M Guidelines Overview◂

►The E/M guidelines have sections that are common to all E/M categories and sections that are category specific. Most of the categories and many of the subcategories of service have special guidelines or instructions unique to that category or subcategory. Where these are indicated, eg, "Inpatient Hospital Care," special instructions are presented before the listing of the specific E/M services codes. It is important to review the instructions for each category or subcategory. These guidelines are to be used by the reporting physician or other qualified health care professional to select the appropriate level of service. These guidelines do not establish documentation requirements or standards of care. The main purpose of documentation is to support care of the patient by current and future health care team(s).

There are two sets of guidelines: one for office or other outpatient services and another for the remaining E/M services. There are sections that are common to both (ie, Guidelines in Common). These guidelines are presented as Guidelines Common to all E/M Services, Guidelines for E/M Services (Hospital Observation, Hospital Inpatient, Consultations, Emergency Department, Nursing Facility, Domiciliary, Rest Home or Custodial Care, Home) and Guidelines for Office or Other Outpatient Services.

The main differences between the two sets of guidelines is that the office or other outpatient services use medical decision making (MDM) ***or*** time as the basis for selecting a code level, whereas the other E/M codes use history, examination, ***and*** MDM and only use time when counseling and/or coordination of care dominates the service. The definitions of time are different for different categories of services.◄

Classification of Evaluation and Management (E/M) Services

►The E/M section is divided into broad categories such as office visits, hospital visits, and consultations. Most of the categories are further divided into two or more subcategories of E/M services. For example, there are two subcategories of office visits (new patient and established patient) and there are two subcategories of hospital visits (initial and subsequent). The subcategories of E/M services are further classified into levels of E/M services that are identified by specific codes.

The basic format of the levels of E/M services is the same for most categories. First, a unique code number is listed. Second, the place and/or type of service is specified, eg, office consultation. Third, the content of the service is defined. Fourth, time is specified. (A detailed discussion of time is provided following the Decision Tree for New vs Established Patients.)◄

►Summary of Guideline Differences◄

►Component(s) for Code Selection	Office or Other Outpatient Services	Other E/M Services (Hospital Observation, Hospital Inpatient, Consultations, Emergency Department, Nursing Facility, Domiciliary, Rest Home, or Custodial Care, Home)
History and Examination	• As medically appropriate. Not used in code selection	• Use key components (history, examination, MDM)
Medical Decision Making (MDM)	• May use MDM or total time on the date of the encounter	• Use key components (history, examination, MDM)
Time	• May use MDM or total time on the date of the encounter	• May use face-to-face time or time at the bedside and on the patient's floor or unit when counseling and/or coordination of care dominates the service. *Time is **not** a descriptive component for the emergency department levels of E/M services.*
MDM Elements	• Number and complexity of problems addressed at the encounter • Amount and/or complexity of data to be reviewed and analyzed • Risk of complications and/or morbidity or mortality of patient management	• Number of diagnoses or management options • Amount and/or complexity of data to be reviewed • Risk of complications and/or morbidity or mortality◄

Definitions of Commonly Used Terms

►Certain key words and phrases are used throughout the E/M section. The following definitions are intended to reduce the potential for differing interpretations and to increase the consistency of reporting by physicians and other qualified health care professionals. The definitions in the E/M section are provided solely for the basis of code selection.

Some definitions are common to all categories of services and others are specific to one or more categories only.◄

►Guidelines Common to All E/M Services◄

►Levels of E/M Services◄

Within each category or subcategory of E/M service, there are three to five levels of E/M services available for reporting purposes. Levels of E/M services are **not** interchangeable among the different categories or subcategories of service. For example, the first level of E/M services in the subcategory of office visit, new patient, does not have the same definition as the first level of E/M services in the subcategory of office visit, established patient. Each level of E/M services may be used by all physicians or other qualified health care professionals.

New and Established Patient

Solely for the purposes of distinguishing between new and established patients, **professional services** are those face-to-face services rendered by physicians and other qualified health care professionals who may report evaluation and management services reported by a specific CPT code(s). A new patient is one who has not received any professional services from the physician/qualified health care professional or another physician/qualified health care professional of the **exact** same specialty **and subspecialty** who belongs to the same group practice, within the past three years.

An established patient is one who has received professional services from the physician/qualified health care professional or another physician/qualified health care professional of the **exact** same specialty **and subspecialty** who belongs to the same group practice, within the past three years. See Decision Tree for New vs Established Patients.

In the instance where a physician/qualified health care professional is on call for or covering for another physician/qualified health care professional, the patient's encounter will be classified as it would have been by the physician/qualified health care professional who is not available. When advanced practice nurses and physician assistants are working with physicians, they are considered as working in the exact same specialty and exact same subspecialties as the physician.

No distinction is made between new and established patients in the emergency department. E/M services in the emergency department category may be reported for any new or established patient who presents for treatment in the emergency department.

The Decision Tree for New vs Established Patients is provided to aid in determining whether to report the E/M service provided as a new or an established patient encounter.

Coding Tip

Instructions for Use of the CPT Codebook

When advanced practice nurses and physician assistants are working with physicians, they are considered as working in the exact same specialty and exact same subspecialties as the physician. A "physician or other qualified health care professional" is an individual who is qualified by education, training, licensure/regulation (when applicable), and facility privileging (when applicable) who performs a professional service within his or her scope of practice and independently reports that professional services. These professionals are distinct from "clinical staff." A clinical staff member is a person who works under the supervision of a physician or other qualified health care professional, and who is allowed by law, regulation and facility policy to perform or assist in the performance of a specific professional service, but does not individually report that professional service. Other policies may also affect who may report specific services.

CPT Coding Guidelines, Introduction, Instructions for Use of the CPT Codebook

Decision Tree for New vs Established Patients

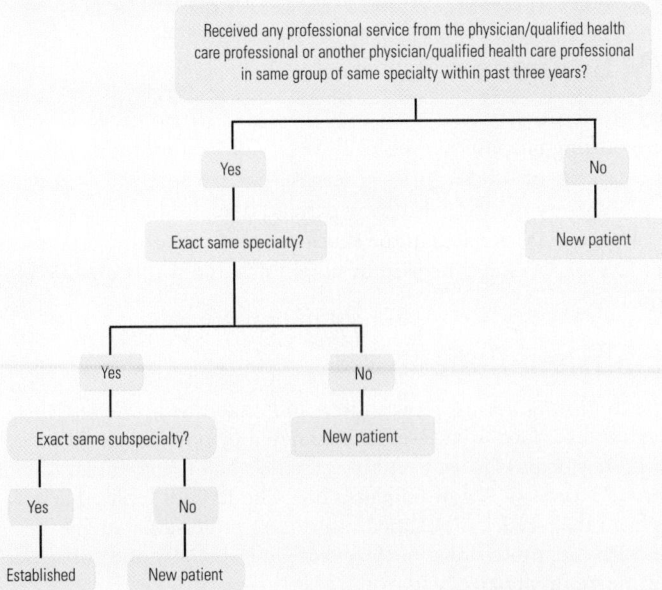

E/M Services Guidelines

Time

►The inclusion of time in the definitions of levels of E/M services has been implicit in prior editions of the CPT codebook. The inclusion of time as an explicit factor beginning in CPT 1992 was done to assist in selecting the most appropriate level of E/M services. Beginning with CPT 2021, except for 99211, time alone may be used to select the appropriate code level for the office or other outpatient E/M services codes (99202, 99203, 99204, 99205, 99212, 99213, 99214, 99215). Different categories of services use time differently. It is important to review the instructions for each category.◄

Time is **not** a descriptive component for the emergency department levels of E/M services because emergency department services are typically provided on a variable intensity basis, often involving multiple encounters with several patients over an extended period of time. Therefore, it is often difficult to provide accurate estimates of the time spent face-to-face with the patient.

►Time may be used to select a code level in office or other outpatient services whether or not counseling and/or coordination of care dominates the service. Time may only be used for selecting the level of the ***other*** E/M services when counseling and/or coordination of care dominates the service.

When time is used for reporting E/M services codes, the time defined in the service descriptors is used for selecting the appropriate level of services. The E/M services for which these guidelines apply require a face-to-face encounter with the physician or other qualified health care professional. For office or other outpatient services, if the physician's or other qualified health care professional's time is spent in the supervision of clinical staff who perform the face-to-face services of the encounter, use 99211.

A shared or split visit is defined as a visit in which a physician and other qualified health care professional(s) jointly provide the face-to-face and non-face-to-face work related to the visit. When time is being used to select the appropriate level of services for which time-based reporting of shared or split visits is allowed, the time personally spent by the physician and other qualified health care professional(s) assessing and managing the patient on the date of the encounter is summed to define total time. Only distinct time should be summed for shared or split visits (ie, when two or more individuals jointly meet with or discuss the patient, only the time of one individual should be counted).

When prolonged time occurs, the appropriate prolonged services code may be reported. The appropriate time should be documented in the medical record when it is used as the basis for code selection.

Face-to-face time (outpatient consultations [99241, 99242, 99243, 99244, 99245], domiciliary, rest home, or custodial services [99324, 99325, 99326, 99327, 99328, 99334, 99335, 99336, 99337], home services [99341, 99342, 99343, 99344, 99345, 99347, 99348, 99349, 99350], cognitive assessment and care plan services [99483]): For coding purposes, face-to-face time for these services is defined as only that time spent face-to-face with the patient and/or family. This includes the time spent performing such tasks as obtaining a history, examination, and counseling the patient.

Unit/floor time (hospital observation services [99218, 99219, 99220, 99224, 99225, 99226, 99234, 99235, 99236], hospital inpatient services [99221, 99222, 99223, 99231, 99232, 99233], inpatient consultations [99251, 99252, 99253, 99254, 99255], nursing facility services [99304, 99305, 99306, 99307, 99308, 99309, 99310, 99315, 99316, 99318]): For coding purposes, time for these services is defined as unit/floor time, which includes the time present on the patient's hospital unit and at the bedside rendering services for that patient. This includes the time to establish and/or review the patient's chart, examine the patient, write notes, and communicate with other professionals and the patient's family.

Total time on the date of the encounter (office or other outpatient services [99202, 99203, 99204, 99205, 99212, 99213, 99214, 99215]): For coding purposes, time for these services is the total time on the date of the encounter. It includes both the face-to-face and non-face-to-face time personally spent by the physician and/or other qualified health care professional(s) on the day of the encounter (includes time in activities that require the physician or other qualified health care professional and does not include time in activities normally performed by clinical staff).

Physician/other qualified health care professional time includes the following activities, when performed:

- preparing to see the patient (eg, review of tests)
- obtaining and/or reviewing separately obtained history
- performing a medically appropriate examination and/or evaluation
- counseling and educating the patient/family/caregiver
- ordering medications, tests, or procedures
- referring and communicating with other health care professionals (when not separately reported)
- documenting clinical information in the electronic or other health record
- independently interpreting results (not separately reported) and communicating results to the patient/family/caregiver
- care coordination (not separately reported)◀

Concurrent Care and Transfer of Care

Concurrent care is the provision of similar services (eg, hospital visits) to the same patient by more than one physician or other qualified health care professional on the same day. When concurrent care is provided, no special reporting is required. Transfer of care is the process whereby a physician or other qualified health care professional who is providing management for some or all of a patient's problems relinquishes this responsibility to another physician or other qualified health care professional who explicitly agrees to accept this responsibility and who, from the initial encounter, is not providing consultative services. The physician or other qualified health care professional transferring care is then no longer providing care for these problems though he or she may continue providing care for other conditions when appropriate. Consultation codes should not be reported by the physician or other qualified health care professional who has agreed to accept transfer of care before an initial evaluation but are appropriate to report if the decision to accept transfer of care cannot be made until after the initial consultation evaluation, regardless of site of service.

Counseling

Counseling is a discussion with a patient and/or family concerning one or more of the following areas:

- Diagnostic results, impressions, and/or recommended diagnostic studies
- Prognosis
- Risks and benefits of management (treatment) options
- Instructions for management (treatment) and/or follow-up
- Importance of compliance with chosen management (treatment) options
- Risk factor reduction
- Patient and family education

(For psychotherapy, see 90832-90834, 90836-90840)

▸Services Reported Separately◂

▶Any specifically identifiable procedure or service (ie, identified with a specific CPT code) performed on the date of E/M services may be reported separately.

The actual performance and/or interpretation of diagnostic tests/studies during a patient encounter are not included in determining the levels of E/M services when reported separately. Physician performance of diagnostic tests/studies for which specific CPT codes are available may be reported separately, in addition to the appropriate E/M code. The physician's interpretation of the results of diagnostic tests/studies (ie, professional component) with preparation of a separate distinctly identifiable signed written report may also be reported separately, using the appropriate CPT code and, if required, with modifier 26 appended. If a test/study is independently interpreted in order to manage the patient as part of the E/M service, but is not separately reported, it is part of MDM.

The physician or other qualified health care professional may need to indicate that on the day a procedure or service identified by a CPT code was performed, the patient's condition required a significant separately identifiable E/M service. The E/M service may be caused or prompted by the symptoms or condition for which the procedure and/or service was provided. This circumstance may be reported by adding modifier 25 to the appropriate level of E/M service. As such, different diagnoses are not required for reporting of the procedure and the E/M services on the same date.◀

▸Guidelines for Hospital Observation, Hospital Inpatient, Consultations, Emergency Department, Nursing Facility, Domiciliary, Rest Home, or Custodial Care, and Home E/M Services◂

Levels of E/M Services

The descriptors for the levels of E/M services recognize seven components, six of which are used in defining the levels of E/M services. These components are:

- History
- Examination
- Medical decision making
- Counseling
- Coordination of care
- Nature of presenting problem
- Time

The first three of these components (history, examination, and medical decision making) are considered the **key** components in selecting a level of E/M services. (See "Determine the Extent of History Obtained.")

The next three components (counseling, coordination of care, and the nature of the presenting problem) are considered **contributory** factors in the majority of encounters. Although the first two of these contributory factors are important E/M services, it is not required that these services be provided at every patient encounter.

Coordination of care with other physicians, other health care professionals, or agencies without a patient encounter on that day is reported using the case management codes.

E/M Services Guidelines

▶The final component, time, is discussed in detail following the Decision Tree for New vs Established Patients.◀

Chief Complaint

A chief complaint is a concise statement describing the symptom, problem, condition, diagnosis, or other factor that is the reason for the encounter, usually stated in the patient's words.

History of Present Illness

A chronological description of the development of the patient's present illness from the first sign and/or symptom to the present. This includes a description of location, quality, severity, timing, context, modifying factors, and associated signs and symptoms significantly related to the presenting problem(s).

Nature of Presenting Problem

A presenting problem is a disease, condition, illness, injury, symptom, sign, finding, complaint, or other reason for encounter, with or without a diagnosis being established at the time of the encounter. The E/M codes recognize five types of presenting problems that are defined as follows:

Minimal: A problem that may not require the presence of the physician or other qualified health care professional, but service is provided under the physician's or other qualified health care professional's supervision.

▶***Self-limited or minor:*** A problem that runs a definite and prescribed course, is transient in nature, and is not likely to permanently alter health status.◀

Low severity: A problem where the risk of morbidity without treatment is low; there is little to no risk of mortality without treatment; full recovery without functional impairment is expected.

Moderate severity: A problem where the risk of morbidity without treatment is moderate; there is moderate risk of mortality without treatment; uncertain prognosis OR increased probability of prolonged functional impairment.

High severity: A problem where the risk of morbidity without treatment is high to extreme; there is a moderate to high risk of mortality without treatment OR high probability of severe, prolonged functional impairment.

Past History

A review of the patient's past experiences with illnesses, injuries, and treatments that includes significant information about:

- Prior major illnesses and injuries
- Prior operations
- Prior hospitalizations
- Current medications
- Allergies (eg, drug, food)
- Age appropriate immunization status
- Age appropriate feeding/dietary status

Family History

A review of medical events in the patient's family that includes significant information about:

- The health status or cause of death of parents, siblings, and children
- Specific diseases related to problems identified in the Chief Complaint or History of the Present Illness, and/or System Review
- Diseases of family members that may be hereditary or place the patient at risk

Social History

An age appropriate review of past and current activities that includes significant information about:

- Marital status and/or living arrangements
- Current employment
- Occupational history
- Military history
- Use of drugs, alcohol, and tobacco
- Level of education
- Sexual history
- Other relevant social factors

System Review (Review of Systems)

An inventory of body systems obtained through a series of questions seeking to identify signs and/or symptoms that the patient may be experiencing or has experienced. For the purposes of the CPT codebook the following elements of a system review have been identified:

- Constitutional symptoms (fever, weight loss, etc)
- Eyes
- Ears, nose, mouth, throat
- Cardiovascular
- Respiratory
- Gastrointestinal
- Genitourinary
- Musculoskeletal
- Integumentary (skin and/or breast)
- Neurological
- Psychiatric
- Endocrine
- Hematologic/lymphatic
- Allergic/immunologic

The review of systems helps define the problem, clarify the differential diagnosis, identify needed testing, or serves as baseline data on other systems that might be affected by any possible management options.

▸Instructions for Selecting a Level of E/M Service for Hospital Observation, Hospital Inpatient, Consultations, Emergency Department, Nursing Facility, Domiciliary, Rest Home, or Custodial Care, and Home E/M Services◂

Review the Level of E/M Service Descriptors and Examples in the Selected Category or Subcategory

The descriptors for the levels of E/M services recognize seven components, six of which are used in defining the levels of E/M services. These components are:

- History
- Examination
- Medical decision making
- Counseling
- Coordination of care
- Nature of presenting problem
- Time

▶The first three of these components (ie, history, examination, and medical decision making) should be considered the **key** components in selecting the level of E/M services. An exception to this rule is in the case of visits that consist predominantly of counseling or coordination of care.◀

The nature of the presenting problem and time are provided in some levels to assist the physician in determining the appropriate level of E/M service.

Determine the Extent of History Obtained

The extent of the history is dependent upon clinical judgment and on the nature of the presenting problem(s). The levels of E/M services recognize four types of history that are defined as follows:

Problem focused: Chief complaint; brief history of present illness or problem.

Expanded problem focused: Chief complaint; brief history of present illness; problem pertinent system review.

Detailed: Chief complaint; extended history of present illness; problem pertinent system review extended to include a review of a limited number of additional systems; **pertinent** past, family, and/or social history **directly related to the patient's problems.**

Comprehensive: Chief complaint; extended history of present illness; review of systems that is directly related to the problem(s) identified in the history of the present illness plus a review of all additional body systems; **complete** past, family, and social history.

The comprehensive history obtained as part of the preventive medicine E/M service is not problem-oriented and does not involve a chief complaint or present illness. It does, however, include a comprehensive system review and comprehensive or interval past, family, and social history as well as a comprehensive assessment/history of pertinent risk factors.

Determine the Extent of Examination Performed

The extent of the examination performed is dependent on clinical judgment and on the nature of the presenting problem(s). The levels of E/M services recognize four types of examination that are defined as follows:

Problem focused: A limited examination of the affected body area or organ system.

Expanded problem focused: A limited examination of the affected body area or organ system and other symptomatic or related organ system(s).

Detailed: An extended examination of the affected body area(s) and other symptomatic or related organ system(s).

Comprehensive: A general multisystem examination or a complete examination of a single organ system. **Note:** The comprehensive examination performed as part of the preventive medicine E/M service is multisystem, but its extent is based on age and risk factors identified.

For the purposes of these CPT definitions, the following body areas are recognized:

- Head, including the face
- Neck
- Chest, including breasts and axilla
- Abdomen
- Genitalia, groin, buttocks
- Back
- Each extremity

For the purposes of these CPT definitions, the following organ systems are recognized:

- Eyes
- Ears, nose, mouth, and throat
- Cardiovascular
- Respiratory
- Gastrointestinal
- Genitourinary
- Musculoskeletal
- Skin
- Neurologic
- Psychiatric
- Hematologic/lymphatic/immunologic

Determine the Complexity of Medical Decision Making

Medical decision making refers to the complexity of establishing a diagnosis and/or selecting a management option as measured by:

- The number of possible diagnoses and/or the number of management options that must be considered
- The amount and/or complexity of medical records, diagnostic tests, and/or other information that must be obtained, reviewed, and analyzed
- The risk of significant complications, morbidity, and/or mortality, as well as comorbidities, associated with the patient's presenting problem(s), the diagnostic procedure(s), and/or the possible management options

Four types of medical decision making are recognized: straightforward, low complexity, moderate complexity, and high complexity. To qualify for a given type of decision making, two of the three elements in Table 1 must be met or exceeded.

E/M Services Guidelines

Table 1
Complexity of Medical Decision Making

Number of Diagnoses or Management Options	Amount and/or Complexity of Data to be Reviewed	Risk of Complications and/or Morbidity or Mortality	Type of Decision Making
minimal	minimal or none	minimal	**straightforward**
limited	limited	low	**low complexity**
multiple	moderate	moderate	**moderate complexity**
extensive	extensive	high	**high complexity**

Comorbidities/underlying diseases, in and of themselves, are not considered in selecting a level of E/M services *unless* their presence significantly increases the complexity of the medical decision making.

Select the Appropriate Level of E/M Services Based on the Following

▶1. For the following categories/subcategories, **all of the key components,** ie, history, examination, and medical decision making, must meet or exceed the stated requirements to qualify for a particular level of E/M service: initial observation care; initial hospital care; observation or inpatient hospital care (including admission and discharge services); office or other outpatient consultations; inpatient consultations; emergency department services; initial nursing facility care; other nursing facility services; domiciliary care, new patient; and home services, new patient.

2. For the following categories/subcategories, **two of the three key components** (ie, history, examination, and medical decision making) must meet or exceed the stated requirements to qualify for a particular level of E/M services: subsequent observation care; subsequent hospital care; subsequent nursing facility care; domiciliary care, established patient; and home services, established patient.◀

3. When counseling and/or coordination of care dominates (more than 50%) the encounter with the patient and/or family (face-to-face time in the office or other outpatient setting or floor/unit time in the hospital or nursing facility), then **time** shall be considered the key or controlling factor to qualify for a particular level of E/M services. This includes time spent with parties who have assumed responsibility for the care of the patient or decision making whether or not they are family members (eg, foster parents, person acting in loco parentis, legal guardian). The extent of counseling and/or coordination of care must be documented in the medical record.

▸Guidelines for Office or Other Outpatient E/M Services◂

▸History and/or Examination◂

▶Office or other outpatient services include a medically appropriate history and/or physical examination, when performed. The nature and extent of the history and/or physical examination are determined by the treating physician or other qualified health care professional reporting the service. The care team may collect information and the patient or caregiver may supply information directly (eg, by electronic health record

[EHR] portal or questionnaire) that is reviewed by the reporting physician or other qualified health care professional. The extent of history and physical examination is not an element in selection of the level of office or other outpatient codes.◀

▸Number and Complexity of Problems Addressed at the Encounter◂

▶One element used in selecting the level of office or other outpatient services is the number and complexity of the problems that are addressed at an encounter. Multiple new or established conditions may be addressed at the same time and may affect MDM. Symptoms may cluster around a specific diagnosis and each symptom is not necessarily a unique condition. Comorbidities/underlying diseases, in and of themselves, are not considered in selecting a level of E/M services **unless** they are addressed, and their presence increases the amount and/or complexity of data to be reviewed and analyzed or the risk of complications and/or morbidity or mortality of patient management. The final diagnosis for a condition does not, in and of itself, determine the complexity or risk, as extensive evaluation may be required to reach the conclusion that the signs or symptoms do not represent a highly morbid condition. Multiple problems of a lower severity may, in the aggregate, create higher risk due to interaction.

Definitions for the elements of MDM (see Table 2, Levels of Medical Decision Making) for other office or other outpatient services are:

Problem: A problem is a disease, condition, illness, injury, symptom, sign, finding, complaint, or other matter addressed at the encounter, with or without a diagnosis being established at the time of the encounter.

Problem addressed: A problem is addressed or managed when it is evaluated or treated at the encounter by the physician or other qualified health care professional reporting the service. This includes consideration of further testing or treatment that may not be elected by virtue of risk/benefit analysis or patient/parent/guardian/surrogate choice. Notation in the patient's medical record that another professional is managing the problem without additional assessment or care coordination documented does not qualify as being addressed or managed by the physician or other qualified health care professional reporting the service. Referral without evaluation (by history, examination, or diagnostic study[ies]) or consideration of treatment does not qualify as being addressed or managed by the physician or other qualified health care professional reporting the service.

Minimal problem: A problem that may not require the presence of the physician or other qualified health care professional, but the service is provided under the physician's or other qualified health care professional's supervision (see 99211).

Self-limited or minor problem: A problem that runs a definite and prescribed course, is transient in nature, and is not likely to permanently alter health status.

Stable, chronic illness: A problem with an expected duration of at least one year or until the death of the patient. For the purpose of defining chronicity, conditions are treated as chronic whether or not stage or severity changes (eg, uncontrolled diabetes and controlled diabetes are a single chronic condition). "Stable" for the purposes of categorizing MDM is defined by the specific treatment goals for an individual patient. A patient who is not at his or her treatment goal is not stable, even if the condition has not changed and there is no short-term threat to life or function. For example, in a patient with persistently poorly controlled blood pressure for whom better control is a goal is not stable, even if the pressures are not changing and the patient is asymptomatic, the risk of morbidity **without** treatment is significant. Examples may include well-controlled hypertension, non-insulin-dependent diabetes, cataract, or benign prostatic hyperplasia.

Acute, uncomplicated illness or injury: A recent or new short-term problem with low risk of morbidity for which treatment is considered. There is little to no risk of mortality with treatment, and full recovery without functional impairment is expected. A problem

E/M Services Guidelines

that is normally self-limited or minor but is not resolving consistent with a definite and prescribed course is an acute, uncomplicated illness. Examples may include cystitis, allergic rhinitis, or a simple sprain.

Chronic illness with exacerbation, progression, or side effects of treatment: A chronic illness that is acutely worsening, poorly controlled, or progressing with an intent to control progression and requiring additional supportive care or requiring attention to treatment for side effects but that does not require consideration of hospital level of care.

Undiagnosed new problem with uncertain prognosis: A problem in the differential diagnosis that represents a condition likely to result in a high risk of morbidity without treatment. An example may be a lump in the breast.

Acute illness with systemic symptoms: An illness that causes systemic symptoms and has a high risk of morbidity without treatment. For systemic general symptoms, such as fever, body aches, or fatigue in a minor illness that may be treated to alleviate symptoms, shorten the course of illness, or to prevent complications, see the definitions for ***self-limited or minor problem*** or ***acute, uncomplicated illness or injury.*** Systemic symptoms may not be general but may be single system. Examples may include pyelonephritis, pneumonitis, or colitis.

Acute, complicated injury: An injury which requires treatment that includes evaluation of body systems that are not directly part of the injured organ, the injury is extensive, or the treatment options are multiple and/or associated with risk of morbidity. An example may be a head injury with brief loss of consciousness.

Chronic illness with severe exacerbation, progression, or side effects of treatment: The severe exacerbation or progression of a chronic illness or severe side effects of treatment that have significant risk of morbidity and may require hospital level of care.

Acute or chronic illness or injury that poses a threat to life or bodily function: An acute illness with systemic symptoms, an acute complicated injury, or a chronic illness or injury with exacerbation and/or progression or side effects of treatment, that poses a threat to life or bodily function in the near term without treatment. Examples may include acute myocardial infarction, pulmonary embolus, severe respiratory distress, progressive severe rheumatoid arthritis, psychiatric illness with potential threat to self or others, peritonitis, acute renal failure, or an abrupt change in neurologic status.

Test: Tests are imaging, laboratory, psychometric, or physiologic data. A clinical laboratory panel (eg, basic metabolic panel [80047]) is a single test. The differentiation between single or multiple unique tests is defined in accordance with the CPT code set.

External: External records, communications and/or test results are from an external physician, other qualified health care professional, facility, or health care organization.

External physician or other qualified health care professional: An external physician or other qualified health care professional who is not in the same group practice or is of a different specialty or subspecialty. This includes licensed professionals who are practicing independently. The individual may also be a facility or organizational provider such as from a hospital, nursing facility, or home health care agency.

Independent historian(s): An individual (eg, parent, guardian, surrogate, spouse, witness) who provides a history in addition to a history provided by the patient who is unable to provide a complete or reliable history (eg, due to developmental stage, dementia, or psychosis) or because a confirmatory history is judged to be necessary. In the case where there may be conflict or poor communication between multiple historians and more than one historian is needed, the independent historian requirement is met.

Independent interpretation: The interpretation of a test for which there is a CPT code and an interpretation or report is customary. This does not apply when the physician or other qualified health care professional is reporting the service or has previously reported the service for the patient. A form of interpretation should be documented but need not conform to the usual standards of a complete report for the test.

Appropriate source: For the purpose of the **discussion of management** data element (see Table 2, Levels of Medical Decision Making), an appropriate source includes professionals who are not health care professionals but may be involved in the management of the patient (eg, lawyer, parole officer, case manager, teacher). It does not include discussion with family or informal caregivers.

Risk: The probability and/or consequences of an event. The assessment of the level of risk is affected by the nature of the event under consideration. For example, a low probability of death may be high risk, whereas a high chance of a minor, self-limited adverse effect of treatment may be low risk. Definitions of risk are based upon the usual behavior and thought processes of a physician or other qualified health care professional in the same specialty. Trained clinicians apply common language usage meanings to terms such as *high, medium, low,* or *minimal* risk and do not require quantification for these definitions (though quantification may be provided when evidence-based medicine has established probabilities). For the purposes of MDM, level of risk is based upon consequences of the problem(s) addressed at the encounter when appropriately treated. Risk also includes MDM related to the need to initiate or forego further testing, treatment, and/or hospitalization.

Morbidity: A state of illness or functional impairment that is expected to be of substantial duration during which function is limited, quality of life is impaired, or there is organ damage that may not be transient despite treatment.

Social determinants of health: Economic and social conditions that influence the health of people and communities. Examples may include food or housing insecurity.

Drug therapy requiring intensive monitoring for toxicity: A drug that requires intensive monitoring is a therapeutic agent that has the potential to cause serious morbidity or death. The monitoring is performed for assessment of these adverse effects and not primarily for assessment of therapeutic efficacy. The monitoring should be that which is generally accepted practice for the agent but may be patient-specific in some cases. Intensive monitoring may be long-term or short-term. Long-term intensive monitoring is not performed less than quarterly. The monitoring may be performed with a laboratory test, a physiologic test, or imaging. Monitoring by history or examination does not qualify. The monitoring affects the level of MDM in an encounter in which it is considered in the management of the patient. Examples may include monitoring for cytopenia in the use of an antineoplastic agent between dose cycles or the short-term intensive monitoring of electrolytes and renal function in a patient who is undergoing diuresis. Examples of monitoring that do not qualify include monitoring glucose levels during insulin therapy, as the primary reason is the therapeutic effect (even if hypoglycemia is a concern); or annual electrolytes and renal function for a patient on a diuretic, as the frequency does not meet the threshold.◀

▸Instructions for Selecting a Level of Office or Other Outpatient E/M Services◂

▶Select the appropriate level of E/M services based on the following:

1. The level of the MDM as defined for each service, **or**
2. The total time for E/M services performed on the date of the encounter.◀

E/M Services Guidelines

▸Medical Decision Making◂

▶MDM includes establishing diagnoses, assessing the status of a condition, and/or selecting a management option. MDM in the office or other outpatient services codes is defined by three elements:

- The number and complexity of problem(s) that are addressed during the encounter.
- The amount and/or complexity of data to be reviewed and analyzed. These data include medical records, tests, and/or other information that must be obtained, ordered, reviewed, and analyzed for the encounter. This includes information obtained from multiple sources or interprofessional communications that are not reported separately and interpretation of tests that are not reported separately. Ordering a test is included in the category of test result(s) and the review of the test result is part of the encounter and not a subsequent encounter. Data are divided into three categories:
  - Tests, documents, orders, or independent historian(s). (Each unique test, order, or document is counted to meet a threshold number.)
  - Independent interpretation of tests.
  - Discussion of management or test interpretation with external physician or other qualified health care professional or appropriate source.
- The risk of complications and/or morbidity or mortality of patient management decisions made at the visit, associated with the patient's problem(s), the diagnostic procedure(s), treatment(s). This includes the possible management options selected and those considered but not selected, after shared MDM with the patient and/or family. For example, a decision about hospitalization includes consideration of alternative levels of care. Examples may include a psychiatric patient with a sufficient degree of support in the outpatient setting or the decision to not hospitalize a patient with advanced dementia with an acute condition that would generally warrant inpatient care, but for whom the goal is palliative treatment.

Four types of MDM are recognized: straightforward, low, moderate, and high. The concept of the level of MDM does not apply to 99211.

Shared MDM involves eliciting patient and/or family preferences, patient and/or family education, and explaining risks and benefits of management options.

MDM may be impacted by role and management responsibility.

When the physician or other qualified health care professional is reporting a separate CPT code that includes interpretation and/or report, the interpretation and/or report should not count toward the MDM when selecting a level of office or other outpatient services. When the physician or other qualified health care professional is reporting a separate service for discussion of management with a physician or another qualified health care professional, the discussion is not counted toward the MDM when selecting a level of office or other outpatient services.

The Levels of Medical Decision Making (MDM) table (Table 2) is a guide to assist in selecting the level of MDM for reporting an office or other outpatient E/M services code. The table includes the four levels of MDM (ie, straightforward, low, moderate, high) and the three elements of MDM (ie, number and complexity of problems addressed at the encounter, amount and/or complexity of data reviewed and analyzed, and risk of complications and/or morbidity or mortality of patient management). To qualify for a particular level of MDM, two of the three elements for that level of MDM must be met or exceeded. See Table 2: Levels of Medical Decision Making (MDM) on the following page. ◀

►Table 2: Levels of Medical Decision Making (MDM)◄

		Elements of Medical Decision Making		
►Code	**Level of MDM** (Based on 2 out of 3 Elements of MDM)	**Number and Complexity of Problems Addressed at the Encounter**	**Amount and/or Complexity of Data to be Reviewed and Analyzed** ****Each unique test, order, or document contributes to the combination of 2 or combination of 3 in Category 1 below.***	**Risk of Complications and/or Morbidity or Mortality of Patient Management**
99211	N/A	N/A	N/A	N/A
99202 **99212**	**Straightforward**	**Minimal** • **1** self-limited or minor problem	**Minimal or none**	**Minimal risk of morbidity from additional diagnostic testing or treatment**
99203 **99213**	**Low**	**Low** • **2** or more self-limited or minor problems; **or** • **1** stable, chronic illness; **or** • **1** acute, uncomplicated illness or injury	**Limited** *(Must meet the requirements of at least 1 of the 2 categories)* **Category 1: Tests and documents** • **Any combination of 2 from the following:** ■ Review of prior external note(s) from each unique source*; ■ Review of the result(s) of each unique test*; ■ Ordering of each unique test* **or** **Category 2: Assessment requiring an independent historian(s)** *(For the categories of independent interpretation of tests and discussion of management or test interpretation, see moderate or high)*	**Low risk of morbidity from additional diagnostic testing or treatment**
99204 **99214**	**Moderate**	**Moderate** • **1** or more chronic illnesses with exacerbation, progression, or side effects of treatment; **or** • **2** or more stable, chronic illnesses; **or** • **1** undiagnosed new problem with uncertain prognosis; **or** • **1** acute illness with systemic symptoms; **or** • **1** acute, complicated injury	**Moderate** *(Must meet the requirements of at least 1 out of 3 categories)* **Category 1: Tests, documents, or independent historian(s)** • **Any combination of 3 from the following:** ■ Review of prior external note(s) from each unique source*; ■ Review of the result(s) of each unique test*; ■ Ordering of each unique test*; ■ Assessment requiring an independent historian(s) **or** **Category 2: Independent interpretation of tests** • Independent interpretation of a test performed by another physician/other qualified health care professional (not separately reported); **or** **Category 3: Discussion of management or test interpretation** • Discussion of management or test interpretation with external physician/other qualified health care professional/appropriate source (not separately reported)	**Moderate risk of morbidity from additional diagnostic testing or treatment** *Examples only:* • Prescription drug management • Decision regarding minor surgery with identified patient or procedure risk factors • Decision regarding elective major surgery without identified patient or procedure risk factors • Diagnosis or treatment significantly limited by social determinants of health

(continued)

▶**Table 2: Levels of Medical Decision Making (MDM)**◀, *continued*

Code	Level of MDM (Based on 2 out of 3 Elements of MDM)	Elements of Medical Decision Making		
		Number and Complexity of Problems Addressed at the Encounter	**Amount and/or Complexity of Data to be Reviewed and Analyzed** ****Each unique test, order, or document contributes to the combination of 2 or combination of 3 in Category 1 below.***	**Risk of Complications and/or Morbidity or Mortality of Patient Management**
99205 **99215**	**High**	**High** • **1** or more chronic illnesses with severe exacerbation, progression, or side effects of treatment; **or** • **1** acute or chronic illness or injury that poses a threat to life or bodily function	**Extensive** *(Must meet the requirements of at least 2 out of 3 categories)* **Category 1: Tests, documents, or independent historian(s)** • **Any combination of 3 from the following:** ▪ Review of prior external note(s) from each unique source*; ▪ Review of the result(s) of each unique test*; ▪ Ordering of each unique test*; ▪ Assessment requiring an independent historian(s) **or** **Category 2: Independent interpretation of tests** • Independent interpretation of a test performed by another physician/other qualified health care professional (not separately reported); **or** **Category 3: Discussion of management or test interpretation** • Discussion of management or test interpretation with external physician/other qualified health care professional/appropriate source (not separately reported)	**High risk of morbidity from additional diagnostic testing or treatment** *Examples only:* • Drug therapy requiring intensive monitoring for toxicity • Decision regarding elective major surgery with identified patient or procedure risk factors • Decision regarding emergency major surgery • Decision regarding hospitalization • Decision not to resuscitate or to de-escalate care because of poor prognosis◀

▸Time◂

▶For instructions on using time to select the level of office or other outpatient E/M services code, see the ***Time*** subsection in the ***Guidelines Common to All E/M Services.***◀

Unlisted Service

An E/M service may be provided that is not listed in this section of the CPT codebook. When reporting such a service, the appropriate unlisted code may be used to indicate the service, identifying it by "Special Report," as discussed in the following paragraph. The "Unlisted Services" and accompanying codes for the E/M section are as follows:

99429 **Unlisted preventive** medicine service

99499 **Unlisted evaluation and management** service

Special Report

An unlisted service or one that is unusual, variable, or new may require a special report demonstrating the medical appropriateness of the service. Pertinent information should include an adequate definition or description of the nature, extent, and need for the procedure and the time, effort, and equipment necessary to provide the service. Additional items that may be included are complexity of symptoms, final diagnosis, pertinent physical findings, diagnostic and therapeutic procedures, concurrent problems, and follow-up care.

Clinical Examples

Clinical examples of the codes for E/M services are provided to assist in understanding the meaning of the descriptors and selecting the correct code. The clinical examples are listed in Appendix C. Each example was developed by the specialties shown.

The same problem, when seen by different specialties, may involve different amounts of work. Therefore, the appropriate level of encounter should be reported using the descriptors rather than the examples.

CHAPTER 6

Evaluation and Management

Office or Other Outpatient Services

The following codes are used to report evaluation and management services provided in the office or in an outpatient or other ambulatory facility. A patient is considered an outpatient until inpatient admission to a health care facility occurs.

To report services provided to a patient who is admitted to a hospital or nursing facility in the course of an encounter in the office or other ambulatory facility, see the notes for initial hospital inpatient care (page 23 [of the *CPT 2021* codebook]) or initial nursing facility care (page 33 [of the *CPT 2021* codebook]).

For services provided in the emergency department, see 99281-99285.

For observation care, see 99217-99226.

For observation or inpatient care services (including admission and discharge services), see 99234-99236.

Coding Tip

Determination of Patient Status as New or Established Patient

Solely for the purposes of distinguishing between new and established patients, **professional services** are those face-to-face services rendered by physicians and other qualified health care professionals who may report evaluation and management services reported by a specific CPT code(s). A new patient is one who has not received any professional services from the physician/qualified health care professional or another physician/qualified health care professional of the **exact** same specialty and subspecialty who belongs to the same group practice, within the past three years.

An established patient is one who has received professional services from the physician/qualified health care professional or another physician/qualified health care professional of the exact same specialty and subspecialty who belongs to the same group practice, within the past three years.

In the instance where a physician/qualified health care professional is on call for or covering for another physician/qualified health care professional, the patient's encounter will be classified as it would have been by the physician/qualified health care professional who is not available. When advanced practice nurses and physician assistants are working with physicians they are considered as working in the **exact** same specialty and exact same **subspecialties** as the physician.

CPT Coding Guidelines, Evaluation and Management, Guidelines Common to All E/M Services, New and Established Patient

New Patient

►(99201 has been deleted. To report, use 99202)◄

★▲ **99202** **Office or other outpatient visit** for the evaluation and management of a new patient, which requires a medically appropriate history and/or examination and straightforward medical decision making.

When using time for code selection, 15-29 minutes of total time is spent on the date of the encounter.

➲ *CPT Changes: An Insider's View* 2013, 2017, 2021

➲ *CPT Assistant* Winter 91:11, Spring 92:13, 24, Summer 92:1, 24, Spring 93:34, Summer 93:2, Fall 93:9, Spring 95:1, Summer 95:4, Fall 95:9, Jul 98:9, Sep 98:5, Feb 00:11, Aug 01:2, Apr 02:14, Oct 04:10, Apr 05:1, 3, Jun 05:11, Dec 05:10, May 06:1, Jun 06:1, Oct 06:15, Apr 07:11, Sep 07:1, Mar 09:3, Aug 09:5, Dec 09:9, Jan 11:3, Mar 12:4, 8, Jan 13:9, Jun 13:3, Aug 13:13, 14, Jan 15:12, Mar 16:11, Sep 16:6, Apr 18:10, Sep 18:14, Jan 19:3, Jan 20:3, Feb 20:3, Mar 20:3

➲ *Clinical Examples in Radiology* Winter 12:9

★▲ **99203** **Office or other outpatient visit** for the evaluation and management of a new patient, which requires a medically appropriate history and/or examination and low level of medical decision making.

When using time for code selection, 30-44 minutes of total time is spent on the date of the encounter.

➲ *CPT Changes: An Insider's View* 2013, 2017, 2021

➲ *CPT Assistant* Winter 91:11, Spring 92:14, 24, Summer 92:1, 24, Spring 93:34, Summer 93:2, Fall 93:9, Spring 95:1, Summer 95:4, Fall 95:9, Jul 98:9, Sep 98:5, Feb 00:11, Aug 01:2, Apr 02:14, Oct 04:10, Feb 05:9, Apr 05:1, 3, Jun 05:11, Dec 05:10, May 06:1, Jun 06:1, Oct 06:15, Apr 07:11, Sep 07:1, Mar 09:3, Aug 09:5, Dec 09:9, Jan 11:3, Mar 12:4, 8, Jan 13:9, Jun 13:3, Aug 13:13, 14, Jan 15:12, Mar 16:11, Sep 16:6, Apr 18:10, Sep 18:14, Jan 19:3, Jan 20:3, Feb 20:3, Mar 20:3

➲ *Clinical Examples in Radiology* Winter 12:9

★▲ **99204** **Office or other outpatient visit** for the evaluation and management of a new patient, which requires a medically appropriate history and/or examination and moderate level of medical decision making.

When using time for code selection, 45-59 minutes of total time is spent on the date of the encounter.

➲ *CPT Changes: An Insider's View* 2013, 2017, 2021

➲ *CPT Assistant* Winter 91:11, Spring 92:14, 24, Summer 92:1, 24, Spring 93:34, Summer 93:2, Fall 93:9, Spring 95:1, Summer 95:4, Fall 95:9, Jul 98:9, Sep 98:5, Feb 00:11, Aug 01:2, Apr 02:14, May 02:1, Oct 04:10, Apr 05:1, 3, Jun 05:11, Dec 05:10, May 06:1, Jun 06:1, Oct 06:15, Apr 07:11, Sep 07:1, Mar 09:3, Aug 09:5, Dec 09:9, Jan 11:3, Mar 12:4, 8, Jan 13:9, Jun 13:3, Aug 13:13, 14, Jan 15:12, Mar 16:11, Sep 16:6, Apr 18:10, Sep 18:14, Jan 19:3, Jan 20:3, Feb 20:3, Mar 20:3

➲ *Clinical Examples in Radiology* Winter 12:9

★▲ **99205** **Office or other outpatient visit** for the evaluation and management of a new patient, which requires a medically appropriate history and/or examination and high level of medical decision making.

When using time for code selection, 60-74 minutes of total time is spent on the date of the encounter.

➲ *CPT Changes: An Insider's View* 2013, 2017, 2021

➲ *CPT Assistant* Winter 91:11, Spring 92:14, 24, Summer 92:1, 24, Spring 93:34, Summer 93:2, Fall 93:9, Spring 95:1, Summer 95:4, Fall 95:9, Jul 98:9, Sep 98:5, Feb 00:11, Aug 01:2, Apr 02:2, May 02:1, Oct 04:10, Apr 05:1, 3, Jun 05:11, Dec 05:10, May 06:1, Jun 06:1, Oct 06:15, Apr 07:11, Sep 07:1, Mar 09:3, Aug 09:5, Dec 09:9, Jul 10:4, Jan 11:3, Jan 12:3, Mar 12:4, 8, Jan 13:9, Jun 13:3, Aug 13:13, 14, Jan 15:12, Mar 16:11, Sep 16:6, Apr 18:10, Sep 18:14, Jan 19:3, Jan 20:3, Feb 20:3, Mar 20:3

➲ *Clinical Examples in Radiology* Winter 12:9

►(For services 75 minutes or longer, use prolonged services code 99417)◄

Established Patient

▲ **99211** **Office or other outpatient visit** for the evaluation and management of an established patient, that may not require the presence of a physician or other qualified health care professional. Usually, the presenting problem(s) are minimal.

➲ *CPT Changes: An Insider's View* 2013, 2021

➲ *CPT Assistant* Winter 91:11, Spring 92:14, 24, Summer 92:1, 24, Spring 93:34, Summer 93:2, Fall 93:9, Spring 95:1, Summer 95:4, Fall 95:9, Oct 96:10, Feb 97:9, May 97:4, Jul 98:9, Sep 98:5, Oct 99:9, Feb 00:11, Aug 01:2, Jan 02:2, Oct 04:10, Feb 05:15, Mar 05:11, Apr 05:1, 3, May 05:1, Jun 05:11, Nov 05:1, Dec 05:10, Feb 06:14, May 06:1, Jun 06:1, Jul 06:19, Oct 06:15, Nov 06:21, Apr 07:11, Jul 07:1, Sep 07:1, Dec 07:9, Mar 08:3, Aug 08:13, Mar 09:3, Aug 09:5, Apr 10:10, Jan 11:3, Jan 12:3, Mar 12:4, 8, Apr 12:10, Jan 13:9, Mar 13:13, Jun 13:3, Aug 13:13, 14, Nov 13:3, Mar 14:14, Jan 15:12, Mar 16:11, Sep 16:6, Mar 17:10, Apr 18:10, Sep 18:14, Jan 19:3, Jan 20:3, Feb 20:3, Mar 20:3

E/M 99202-99499

★▲ **99212** **Office or other outpatient visit** for the evaluation and management of an established patient, which requires a medically appropriate history and/or examination and straightforward medical decision making.

When using time for code selection, 10-19 minutes of total time is spent on the date of the encounter.

➲ *CPT Changes: An Insider's View* 2013, 2017, 2021

➲ *CPT Assistant* Winter 91:11, Spring 92:14, 24, Summer 92:1, 24, Spring 93:34, Summer 93:2, Fall 93:9, Spring 95:1, Summer 95:4, Fall 95:9, Jul 98:9, Sep 98:5, Feb 00:11, Jun 00:11, Aug 01:2, Jan 02:2, May 02:3, Apr 04:14, Oct 04:10, Apr 05:1, 3, Jun 05:11, Dec 05:10, May 06:1, Jun 06:1, 11, Sep 06:8, Oct 06:15, Apr 07:11, Jul 07:1, Sep 07:1, Mar 08:3, Mar 09:3, Aug 09:5, Feb 10:13, Jul 10:4, Sep 10:4, Jan 11:3, Jun 11:3, Mar 12:4, 8, Apr 12:17, Jan 13:9, Mar 13:13, Jun 13:3, Aug 13:13, 14, Feb 14:11, Jan 15:12, Mar 16:11, Sep 16:6, Dec 16:12, Oct 17:6, Apr 18:10, Sep 18:14, Jan 19:3, Jan 20:3, Feb 20:3, Mar 20:3

★▲ **99213** **Office or other outpatient visit** for the evaluation and management of an established patient, which requires a medically appropriate history and/or examination and low level of medical decision making.

When using time for code selection, 20-29 minutes of total time is spent on the date of the encounter.

➲ *CPT Changes: An Insider's View* 2013, 2017, 2021

➲ *CPT Assistant* Winter 91:11, Spring 92:14, 24, Summer 92:1, 24, Spring 93:34, Summer 93:2, Fall 93:9, Spring 95:1, Summer 95:4, Fall 95:9, Jan 97:10, Jul 98:9, Sep 98:5, Aug 01:2, May 02:3, Oct 03:5, Apr 04:14, Oct 04:10, Mar 05:11, Apr 05:1, 3, Jun 05:11, Dec 05:10, May 06:1, Jun 06:1, 11, Sep 06:8, Oct 06:15, Apr 07:11, Jul 07:1, Sep 07:1, Mar 08:3, Mar 09:3, Aug 09:5, Sep 10:4, Jan 11:3, Jun 11:3, Mar 12:4, 8, Jan 13:9, Mar 13:13, Jun 13:3, Aug 13:13, 14, Jan 15:12, Mar 16:11, Sep 16:6, Apr 18:10, Sep 18:14, Jan 19:3, Jan 20:3, Feb 20:3, Mar 20:3

★▲ **99214** **Office or other outpatient visit** for the evaluation and management of an established patient, which requires a medically appropriate history and/or examination and moderate level of medical decision making.

When using time for code selection, 30-39 minutes of total time is spent on the date of the encounter.

➲ *CPT Changes: An Insider's View* 2013, 2017, 2021

➲ *CPT Assistant* Winter 91:11, Spring 92:15, 24, Summer 92:1, 24, Spring 93:34, Summer 93:2, Fall 93:9, Spring 95:1, Summer 95:4, Fall 95:9, May 97:4, Jul 98:9, Sep 98:5, Aug 01:2, Jan 02:2, May 02:1-2, Oct 03:5, Apr 04:14, Oct 04:10, Apr 05:1, 3, Jun 05:11, Dec 05:10, May 06:1, Jun 06:1, 11, Sep 06:8, Oct 06:15, Apr 07:11, Jul 07:1, Sep 07:1, Mar 08:3, Mar 09:3, Aug 09:5, Sep 10:4, Jan 11:3, Jun 11:3, Mar 12:4, 8, Jan 13:9, Mar 13:13, Jun 13:3, Aug 13:13, 14, Jan 15:12, Oct 15:3, Mar 16:11, Sep 16:6, Apr 18:10, Sep 18:14, Jan 19:3, Jan 20:3, Feb 20:3, Mar 20:3

★▲ **99215** **Office or other outpatient visit** for the evaluation and management of an established patient, which requires a medically appropriate history and/or examination and high level of medical decision making.

When using time for code selection, 40-54 minutes of total time is spent on the date of the encounter.

➲ *CPT Changes: An Insider's View* 2013, 2017, 2021

➲ *CPT Assistant* Winter 91:11, Spring 92:15, 24, Summer 92:1, 24, Spring 93:34, Summer 93:2, Fall 93:9, Spring 95:1, Summer 95:4, Fall 95:9, Jan 97:10, Jul 98:9, Sep 98:5, Aug 01:2, Jan 02:2, May 02:1, 3, Apr 04:14, Oct 04:10, Mar 05:11, Apr 05:1, 3, Jun 05:11, Dec 05:10, May 06:1, Jun 06:1, 11, Sep 06:8, Oct 06:15, Apr 07:11, Jul 07:1, Sep 07:1, Mar 08:3, Mar 09:3, Aug 09:5, Jul 10:4, Sep 10:4, Jan 11:3, Jun 11:3, Jan 12:3, Mar 12:4, 8, Apr 12:10, Jan 13:9, Mar 13:13, Jun 13:3, Aug 13:13, 14, Nov 13:3, Aug 14:3, Oct 14:3, Nov 14:14, Jan 15:12, Mar 16:11, Sep 16:6, Apr 18:10, Sep 18:14, Jan 19:3, Oct 19:10, Jan 20:3, Feb 20:3, Mar 20:3

►(For services 55 minutes or longer, use prolonged services code 99417)◄

Hospital Observation Services

The following codes are used to report evaluation and management services provided to patients designated/admitted as "observation status" in a hospital. It is not necessary that the patient be located in an observation area designated by the hospital.

If such an area does exist in a hospital (as a separate unit in the hospital, in the emergency department, etc.), these codes are to be utilized if the patient is placed in such an area.

For definitions of key components and commonly used terms, please see **Evaluation and Management Services Guidelines.**

Coding Tip

The Significance of Time as a Factor in Selection of an Evaluation and Management Code from This Section

The inclusion of time as an explicit factor beginning in CPT 1992 was done to assist in selecting the most appropriate level of E/M services included in codes in this section. Beginning with CPT 2021, except for 99211, time alone may be used to select the appropriate code level for the office or other outpatient E/M services codes (99202, 99203, 99204, 99205, 99212, 99213, 99214, 99215). Different categories of services use time differently. It is important to review the instructions for each category.

Unit/floor time (hospital observation services [99218, 99219, 99220, 99224, 99225, 99226, 99234, 99235, 99236], hospital inpatient services [99221, 99222, 99223, 99231, 99232, 99233], inpatient consultations [99251, 99252, 99253, 99254, 99255], nursing facility services [99304, 99305, 99306, 99307, 99308, 99309, 99310, 99315, 99316, 99318]):

For coding purposes, time for these services is defined as unit/floor time, which includes the time present on the patient's hospital unit and at the bedside rendering services for that patient. This includes the time to establish and/or review the patient's chart, examine the patient, write notes, and communicate with other professionals and the patient's family.

CPT Coding Guidelines, Evaluation and Management, Guidelines Common to All E/M Services, Time

Observation Care Discharge Services

Observation care discharge of a patient from "observation status" includes final examination of the patient, discussion of the hospital stay, instructions for continuing care, and preparation of discharge records. For observation or inpatient hospital care including the admission and discharge of the patient on the same date, see codes 99234-99236 as appropriate.

99217 **Observation care discharge** day management (This code is to be utilized to report all services provided to a patient on discharge from outpatient hospital "observation status" if the discharge is on other than the initial date of "observation status." To report services to a patient designated as "observation status" or "inpatient status" and discharged on the same date, use the codes for Observation or Inpatient Care Services [including Admission and Discharge Services, 99234-99236 as appropriate.])

➔ *CPT Changes: An Insider's View* 2013, 2018

➔ *CPT Assistant* Nov 97:2, Mar 98:1, May 98:3, Sep 98:5, Sep 00:3, May 05:1, Nov 05:10, Sep 06:8, Dec 06:14, Sep 10:4, Jun 11:3, Jul 12:10, 11, 14, Jan 13:9, Jun 13:3, Nov 14:14, Jul 19:10

Initial Observation Care

New or Established Patient

The following codes are used to report the encounter(s) by the supervising physician or other qualified health care professional with the patient when designated as outpatient hospital "observation status." This refers to the initiation of observation status, supervision of the care plan for observation and performance of periodic reassessments. For observation encounters by other physicians, see office or other outpatient consultation codes (99241-99245) or subsequent observation care codes (99224-99226) as appropriate.

To report services provided to a patient who is admitted to the hospital after receiving hospital observation care services on the same date, see the notes for initial hospital inpatient care (page 23 [of the *CPT 2021* codebook]). For observation care services on other than the initial or discharge date, see subsequent observation services codes (99224-99226). For a patient admitted to the hospital on a date subsequent to the date of observation status, the hospital admission would be reported with the appropriate initial hospital care code (99221-99223). For a patient admitted and discharged from observation or inpatient status on the same date, the services should be reported with codes 99234-99236 as appropriate. Do not report observation discharge (99217) in conjunction with a hospital admission (99221-99223).

When "observation status" is initiated in the course of an encounter in another site of service (eg, hospital emergency department, office, nursing facility) all evaluation and management services provided by the supervising physician or other qualified health care professional in conjunction with initiating "observation status" are considered part of the initial observation care when performed on the same date. The observation care level of service reported by the supervising physician or other qualified health care professional should include the services related to initiating "observation status" provided in the other sites of service as well as in the observation setting.

▶Evaluation and management services including new or established patient office or other outpatient services (99202-99215), emergency department services (99281-99285), nursing facility services (99304-99318), domiciliary, rest home, or custodial care services (99324-99337), home services (99341-99350), and preventive medicine services (99381-99429) on the same date related to the admission to "observation status" should not be reported separately.◀

These codes may not be utilized for post-operative recovery if the procedure is considered part of the surgical "package." These codes apply to all evaluation and management services that are provided on the same date of initiating "observation status."

99218 **Initial observation care,** per day, for the evaluation and management of a patient which requires these 3 key components:

- **A detailed or comprehensive history;**
- **A detailed or comprehensive examination; and**
- **Medical decision making that is straightforward or of low complexity.**

Counseling and/or coordination of care with other physicians, other qualified health care professionals, or agencies are provided consistent with the nature of the problem(s) and the patient's and/or family's needs.

Usually, the problem(s) requiring admission to outpatient hospital "observation status" are of low severity. Typically, 30 minutes are spent at the bedside and on the patient's hospital floor or unit.

➲ *CPT Changes: An Insider's View* 2012, 2013, 2018

➲ *CPT Assistant* Spring 93:34, Fall 95:9, Nov 97:2, Mar 98:1, Sep 98:5, Sep 00:3, Jan 03:10, Aug 04:11, May 05:1, Nov 05:10, Sep 06:8, Dec 06:14, Sep 10:4, Oct 10:6, Jun 11:3, Jul 12:11, 14, Jan 13:9, Jun 13:3, Aug 13:13, Mar 15:3, Jul 15:3, Dec 18:8, Jul 19:10

E/M 99202-99499

99219 **Initial observation care,** per day, for the evaluation and management of a patient, which requires these 3 key components:

- **A comprehensive history;**
- **A comprehensive examination; and**
- **Medical decision making of moderate complexity.**

Counseling and/or coordination of care with other physicians, other qualified health care professionals, or agencies are provided consistent with the nature of the problem(s) and the patient's and/or family's needs.

Usually, the problem(s) requiring admission to outpatient hospital "observation status" are of moderate severity. Typically, 50 minutes are spent at the bedside and on the patient's hospital floor or unit.

➲ *CPT Changes: An Insider's View* 2012, 2013, 2018

➲ *CPT Assistant* Spring 93:34, Fall 95:16, Nov 97:2, Mar 98:1, Sep 98:5, Sep 00:3, Jan 03:10, Aug 04:11, Nov 05:10, Sep 06:8, Dec 06:14, Sep 10:4, Oct 10:6, Jun 11:3, Jul 12:11, 14, Jan 13:9, Jun 13:3, Aug 13:13, Dec 18:8, Jul 19:10

99220 **Initial observation care,** per day, for the evaluation and management of a patient, which requires these 3 key components:

- **A comprehensive history;**
- **A comprehensive examination; and**
- **Medical decision making of high complexity.**

Counseling and/or coordination of care with other physicians, other qualified health care professionals, or agencies are provided consistent with the nature of the problem(s) and the patient's and/or family's needs.

Usually, the problem(s) requiring admission to outpatient hospital "observation status" are of high severity. Typically, 70 minutes are spent at the bedside and on the patient's hospital floor or unit.

➲ *CPT Changes: An Insider's View* 2012, 2013, 2018

➲ *CPT Assistant* Spring 93:34, Fall 95:16, Nov 97:2, Mar 98:1, Sep 98:5, Sep 00:3, Jan 03:10, Aug 04:11, Nov 05:10, Sep 06:8, Dec 06:14, Sep 10:4, Oct 10:6, Jun 11:3, Jul 12:11, Jan 13:9, Jun 13:3, Aug 13:13, Nov 14:14, Dec 18:8, Jul 19:10

Subsequent Observation Care

All levels of subsequent observation care include reviewing the medical record and reviewing the results of diagnostic studies and changes in the patient's status (ie, changes in history, physical condition, and response to management) since the last assessment.

 # 99224 **Subsequent observation care,** per day, for the evaluation and management of a patient, which requires at least 2 of these 3 key components:

- **Problem focused interval history;**
- **Problem focused examination;**
- **Medical decision making that is straightforward or of low complexity.**

Counseling and/or coordination of care with other physicians, other qualified health care professionals, or agencies are provided consistent with the nature of the problem(s) and the patient's and/or family's needs.

Usually, the patient is stable, recovering, or improving. Typically, 15 minutes are spent at the bedside and on the patient's hospital floor or unit.

➲ *CPT Changes: An Insider's View* 2011, 2013

➲ *CPT Assistant* Jun 11:3, Aug 11:11, Jul 12:10, 11, Jun 13:3, Aug 13:13, Nov 14:14, Jul 19:10

 # 99225 **Subsequent observation care,** per day, for the evaluation and management of a patient, which requires at least 2 of these 3 key components:

- **An expanded problem focused interval history;**
- **An expanded problem focused examination;**
- **Medical decision making of moderate complexity.**

Counseling and/or coordination of care with other physicians, other qualified health care professionals, or agencies are provided consistent with the nature of the problem(s) and the patient's and/or family's needs.

Usually, the patient is responding inadequately to therapy or has developed a minor complication. Typically, 25 minutes are spent at the bedside and on the patient's hospital floor or unit.

CPT Changes: An Insider's View 2011, 2013

CPT Assistant Jun 11:3, Aug 11:11, Jul 12:10, 11, Jan 13:9, Jun 13:3, Aug 13:13, Jul 19:10

 # 99226 **Subsequent observation care,** per day, for the evaluation and management of a patient, which requires at least 2 of these 3 key components:

- **A detailed interval history;**
- **A detailed examination;**
- **Medical decision making of high complexity.**

Counseling and/or coordination of care with other physicians, other qualified health care professionals, or agencies are provided consistent with the nature of the problem(s) and the patient's and/or family's needs.

Usually, the patient is unstable or has developed a significant complication or a significant new problem. Typically, 35 minutes are spent at the bedside and on the patient's hospital floor or unit.

CPT Changes: An Insider's View 2011, 2013

CPT Assistant Jun 11:3, Aug 11:11, Jul 12:10, 11, Jan 13:9, Jun 13:3, Aug 13:13, Nov 14:14, Jul 19:10

Hospital Inpatient Services

The following codes are used to report evaluation and management services provided to hospital inpatients. Hospital inpatient services include those services provided to patients in a "partial hospital" setting. These codes are to be used to report these partial hospitalization services. See also psychiatry notes in the full text of the CPT code set.

For definitions of key components and commonly used terms, see **Evaluation and Management Services Guidelines.** For Hospital Observation Services, see 99218-99220, 99224-99226. For a patient admitted and discharged from observation or inpatient status on the same date, the services should be reported with codes 99234-99236 as appropriate.

E/M 99202-99499

Coding Tip

The Significance of Time as a Factor in Selection of an Evaluation and Management Code from This Section

The inclusion of time as an explicit factor beginning in CPT 1992 was done to assist in selecting the most appropriate level of E/M services included in codes in this section. Beginning with CPT 2021, except for 99211, time alone may be used to select the appropriate code level for the office or other outpatient E/M services codes (99202, 99203, 99204, 99205, 99212, 99213, 99214, 99215). Different categories of services use time differently. It is important to review the instructions for each category.

Unit/floor time (hospital observation services [99218, 99219, 99220, 99224, 99225, 99226, 99234, 99235, 99236], hospital inpatient services [99221, 99222, 99223, 99231, 99232, 99233], inpatient consultations [99251, 99252, 99253, 99254, 99255], nursing facility services [99304, 99305, 99306, 99307, 99308, 99309, 99310, 99315, 99316, 99318]):

For coding purposes, time for these services is defined as unit/floor time, which includes the time present on the patient's hospital unit and at the bedside rendering services for that patient. This includes the time to establish and/or review the patient's chart, examine the patient, write notes, and communicate with other professionals and the patient's family.

CPT Coding Guidelines, Evaluation and Management, Guidelines Common to All E/M Services, Time

Initial Hospital Care

New or Established Patient

The following codes are used to report the first hospital inpatient encounter with the patient by the admitting physician.

For initial inpatient encounters by physicians other than the admitting physician, see initial inpatient consultation codes (99251-99255) or subsequent hospital care codes (99231-99233) as appropriate.

For admission services for the neonate (28 days of age or younger) requiring intensive observation, frequent interventions, and other intensive care services, see 99477.

When the patient is admitted to the hospital as an inpatient in the course of an encounter in another site of service (eg, hospital emergency department, observation status in a hospital, office, nursing facility) all evaluation and management services provided by that physician in conjunction with that admission are considered part of the initial hospital care when performed on the same date as the admission. The inpatient care level of service reported by the admitting physician should include the services related to the admission he/she provided in the other sites of service as well as in the inpatient setting.

►Evaluation and management services including new or established patient office or other outpatient services (99202-99215), emergency department services (99281-99285), nursing facility services (99304-99318), domiciliary, rest home, or custodial care services (99324-99337), home services (99341-99350), and preventive medicine services (99381-99397) on the same date related to the admission to "observation status" should **not** be reported separately. For a patient admitted and discharged from observation or inpatient status on the same date, the services should be reported with codes 99234-99236 as appropriate.◄

99221 **Initial hospital care,** per day, for the evaluation and management of a patient, which requires these 3 key components:

- **A detailed or comprehensive history;**
- **A detailed or comprehensive examination; and**
- **Medical decision making that is straightforward or of low complexity.**

Counseling and/or coordination of care with other physicians, other qualified health care professionals, or agencies are provided consistent with the nature of the problem(s) and the patient's and/or family's needs.

Usually, the problem(s) requiring admission are of low severity. Typically, 30 minutes are spent at the bedside and on the patient's hospital floor or unit.

➲ *CPT Changes: An Insider's View* 2013

➲ *CPT Assistant* Winter 91:11, Spring 92:14, 24, Summer 92:10, 24, Fall 92:1, Spring 93:34, Spring 95:1, Fall 95:9, Jul 96:11, Sep 96:10, Nov 97:2, Mar 98:1, Sep 98:5, Jan 02:2-3, Apr 03:26, Apr 04:14, Aug 04:11, May 05:1, Sep 06:8, Jul 07:12, Jul 12:12, Jan 13:9, Jun 13:3, Aug 13:13, Feb 14:11, May 14:4, Nov 14:14, Dec 15:16, Mar 16:11, Dec 18:8

E/M 99202-99499

99222 **Initial hospital care,** per day, for the evaluation and management of a patient, which requires these 3 key components:

- **A comprehensive history;**
- **A comprehensive examination; and**
- **Medical decision making of moderate complexity.**

Counseling and/or coordination of care with other physicians, other qualified health care professionals, or agencies are provided consistent with the nature of the problem(s) and the patient's and/or family's needs.

Usually, the problem(s) requiring admission are of moderate severity. Typically, 50 minutes are spent at the bedside and on the patient's hospital floor or unit.

➲ *CPT Changes: An Insider's View* 2013

➲ *CPT Assistant* Winter 91:11, Spring 92:14, 24, Summer 92:10, 24, Fall 92:1, Spring 93:34, Spring 95:1, Fall 95:9, Jul 96:11, Sep 96:10, Nov 97:2, Mar 98:1, Sep 98:5, Jan 02:2-3, Apr 03:26, Apr 04:14, Aug 04:11, Sep 06:8, Jul 07:12, Jul 12:12, Jan 13:9, Jun 13:3, Aug 13:13, Mar 15:3, Dec 15:16, Mar 16:11, Dec 18:8

99223 **Initial hospital care,** per day, for the evaluation and management of a patient, which requires these 3 key components:

- **A comprehensive history;**
- **A comprehensive examination; and**
- **Medical decision making of high complexity.**

Counseling and/or coordination of care with other physicians, other qualified health care professionals, or agencies are provided consistent with the nature of the problem(s) and the patient's and/or family's needs.

Usually, the problem(s) requiring admission are of high severity. Typically, 70 minutes are spent at the bedside and on the patient's hospital floor or unit.

➲ *CPT Changes: An Insider's View* 2013

➲ *CPT Assistant* Winter 91:11, Spring 92:14, 24, Summer 92:10, 24, Fall 92:1, Spring 93:34, Spring 95:1, Fall 95:9, Jul 96:11, Sep 96:10, Nov 97:2, Mar 98:1, Sep 98:5, Jan 02:2-3, Apr 03:26, Apr 04:14, Aug 04:11, Sep 06:8, Jul 07:12, Jul 12:12, Jan 13:9, Jun 13:3, Aug 13:13, May 14:4, Nov 14:14, Dec 15:16, Mar 16:11, Dec 18:8

99224 Code is out of numerical sequence. See 99219-99222

99225 Code is out of numerical sequence. See 99219-99222

99226 Code is out of numerical sequence. See 99219-99222

Subsequent Hospital Care

All levels of subsequent hospital care include reviewing the medical record and reviewing the results of diagnostic studies and changes in the patient's status (ie, changes in history, physical condition and response to management) since the last assessment.

★ **99231** **Subsequent hospital care,** per day, for the evaluation and management of a patient, which requires at least 2 of these 3 key components:

- **A problem focused interval history;**
- **A problem focused examination;**
- **Medical decision making that is straightforward or of low complexity.**

Counseling and/or coordination of care with other physicians, other qualified health care professionals, or agencies are provided consistent with the nature of the problem(s) and the patient's and/or family's needs.

Usually, the patient is stable, recovering or improving. Typically, 15 minutes are spent at the bedside and on the patient's hospital floor or unit.

➲ *CPT Changes: An Insider's View* 2013, 2017

➲ *CPT Assistant* Winter 91:11, Spring 92:14, 24, Summer 92:10, 24, Fall 92:1, Spring 93:34, Spring 95:1, Fall 95:16, Nov 97:2, Sep 98:5, Jan 99:10, Nov 99:5, Aug 01:2, Jan 02:2-3, Apr 04:14, Aug 04:11, Mar 05:11, May 05:1, May 06:1, 16, Jul 06:4, Mar 07:9, Jul 07:1, Mar 09:3, Dec 09:9, Jun 11:3, Jul 12:12, Jan 13:9, Jun 13:3, Aug 13:14, Sep 13:18, May 14:4, Nov 14:14, Dec 18:8

★ **99232** **Subsequent hospital care,** per day, for the evaluation and management of a patient, which requires at least 2 of these 3 key components:

- **An expanded problem focused interval history;**
- **An expanded problem focused examination;**
- **Medical decision making of moderate complexity.**

Counseling and/or coordination of care with other physicians, other qualified health care professionals, or agencies are provided consistent with the nature of the problem(s) and the patient's and/or family's needs.

Usually, the patient is responding inadequately to therapy or has developed a minor complication. Typically, 25 minutes are spent at the bedside and on the patient's hospital floor or unit.

➲ *CPT Changes: An Insider's View* 2013, 2017

➲ *CPT Assistant* Winter 91:11, Spring 92:14, 24, Summer 92:10, 24, Fall 92:1, Spring 93:34, Spring 95:1, Fall 95:16, Nov 97:2, Sep 98:5, Jan 99:10, Nov 99:5, Jan 00:11, Aug 01:2, Apr 04:14, Aug 04:11, May 06:1, 16, Jul 06:4, Mar 07:9, Jul 07:1, Mar 09:3, Dec 09:9, Jun 11:3, Jul 12:12, Jan 13:9, Jun 13:3, Aug 13:14, Oct 16:8, Dec 18:8

★ **99233** **Subsequent hospital care,** per day, for the evaluation and management of a patient, which requires at least 2 of these 3 key components:

- **A detailed interval history;**
- **A detailed examination;**
- **Medical decision making of high complexity.**

Counseling and/or coordination of care with other physicians, other qualified health care professionals, or agencies are provided consistent with the nature of the problem(s) and the patient's and/or family's needs.

Usually, the patient is unstable or has developed a significant complication or a significant new problem. Typically, 35 minutes are spent at the bedside and on the patient's hospital floor or unit.

➲ *CPT Changes: An Insider's View* 2013, 2017

➲ *CPT Assistant* Winter 91:11, Spring 92:14, 24, Summer 92:10, 24, Fall 92:1, Spring 93:34, Spring 95:1, Fall 95:16, Nov 97:2, Sep 98:5, Jan 99:10, Nov 99:5, Aug 01:2, Apr 04:14, Aug 04:11, May 06:1, 16, Jul 06:4, Mar 07:9, Jul 07:1, Mar 09:3, Dec 09:9, Jun 11:3, Jul 12:12, Jan 13:9, Jun 13:3, Aug 13:13, 14, May 14:4, Nov 14:14, Oct 16:8, Dec 18:8

Observation or Inpatient Care Services (Including Admission and Discharge Services)

The following codes are used to report observation or inpatient hospital care services provided to patients admitted and discharged on the same date of service. When a patient is admitted to the hospital from observation status on the same date, only the initial hospital care code should be reported. The initial hospital care code reported by the admitting physician or other qualified health care professional should include the services related to the observation status services he/she provided on the same date of inpatient admission.

When "observation status" is initiated in the course of an encounter in another site of service (eg, hospital emergency department, office, nursing facility) all evaluation and management services provided by the supervising physician or other qualified health care professional in conjunction with initiating "observation status" are considered part of the initial observation care when performed on the same date. The observation care level of service should include the services related to initiating "observation status" provided in the other sites of service as well as in the observation setting when provided by the same individual.

For patients admitted to observation or inpatient care and discharged on a different date, see codes 99217, 99218-99220, 99224-99226, or 99221-99223, 99238 and 99239.

99234 **Observation or inpatient hospital care,** for the evaluation and management of a patient including admission and discharge on the same date, which requires these 3 key components:

- **A detailed or comprehensive history;**
- **A detailed or comprehensive examination; and**
- **Medical decision making that is straightforward or of low complexity.**

Counseling and/or coordination of care with other physicians, other qualified health care professionals, or agencies are provided consistent with the nature of the problem(s) and the patient's and/or family's needs.

Usually the presenting problem(s) requiring admission are of low severity. Typically, 40 minutes are spent at the bedside and on the patient's hospital floor or unit.

➲ *CPT Changes: An Insider's View* 2013

➲ *CPT Assistant* Nov 97:2, Mar 98:2, May 98:1, Sep 98:5, Jan 00:11, Sep 00:3, Jan 02:2, Jun 02:10, Jan 03:10, May 05:1, Nov 05:10, Sep 06:8, Dec 06:14, Sep 10:4, Jun 11:3, Jul 12:14, Jun 13:3, Apr 18:10, Dec 18:8

99235 **Observation or inpatient hospital care,** for the evaluation and management of a patient including admission and discharge on the same date, which requires these 3 key components:

- **A comprehensive history;**
- **A comprehensive examination; and**
- **Medical decision making of moderate complexity.**

Counseling and/or coordination of care with other physicians, other qualified health care professionals, or agencies are provided consistent with the nature of the problem(s) and the patient's and/or family's needs.

Usually the presenting problem(s) requiring admission are of moderate severity. Typically, 50 minutes are spent at the bedside and on the patient's hospital floor or unit.

➲ *CPT Changes: An Insider's View* 2013

➲ *CPT Assistant* Nov 97:2, Mar 98:2, May 98:1, Sep 98:5, Jan 00:11, Sep 00:3, Jan 02:2, Jun 02:10, Jan 03:10, Nov 05:10, Sep 06:8, Dec 06:14, Sep 10:4, Jun 11:3, Jul 12:14, Jun 13:3, Apr 18:10, Dec 18:8

99236 **Observation or inpatient hospital care,** for the evaluation and management of a patient including admission and discharge on the same date, which requires these 3 key components:

- **A comprehensive history;**
- **A comprehensive examination; and**
- **Medical decision making of high complexity.**

Counseling and/or coordination of care with other physicians, other qualified health care professionals, or agencies are provided consistent with the nature of the problem(s) and the patient's and/or family's needs.

Usually the presenting problem(s) requiring admission are of high severity. Typically, 55 minutes are spent at the bedside and on the patient's hospital floor or unit.

➲ *CPT Changes: An Insider's View* 2013

➲ *CPT Assistant* Nov 97:2, Mar 98:2, May 98:1, Sep 98:5, Jan 00:11, Sep 00:3, Jan 02:2, Jun 02:10, Jan 03:10, Nov 05:10, Sep 06:8, Dec 06:14, Sep 10:4, Jun 11:3, Jul 12:14, Jun 13:3, Apr 18:10, Dec 18:8

Hospital Discharge Services

The hospital discharge day management codes are to be used to report the total duration of time spent by a physician for final hospital discharge of a patient. The codes include, as appropriate, final examination of the patient, discussion of the hospital stay, even if the time spent by the physician on that date is not continuous, instructions for continuing care to all relevant caregivers, and preparation of discharge records, prescriptions and referral forms. For a patient admitted and discharged from observation or inpatient status on the same date, the services should be reported with codes 99234-99236 as appropriate.

99238 **Hospital discharge day management**; 30 minutes or less

CPT Assistant Fall 92:1, Spring 93:4, Nov 97:4, Mar 98:3, 11, May 98:2, Jan 99:10, Jan 02:2, Aug 04:11, May 05:1, Sep 06:8, Nov 09:10, Dec 09:9, Jul 11:16, Jul 12:10, 12, Jun 13:3, Aug 13:13, Dec 18:8

99239 more than 30 minutes

CPT Assistant Nov 97:4, Mar 98:3, 11, May 98:2, Jan 99:10, Jan 02:2, Aug 04:11, Sep 06:8, Nov 09:10, Dec 09:9, Jul 11:16, Jul 12:12, Jun 13:3, Aug 13:13, Dec 18:8

(These codes are to be utilized to report all services provided to a patient on the date of discharge, if other than the initial date of inpatient status. To report services to a patient who is admitted as an inpatient and discharged on the same date, see codes 99234-99236 for observation or inpatient hospital care including the admission and discharge of the patient on the same date. To report concurrent care services provided by an individual other than the physician or qualified health care professional performing the discharge day management service, use subsequent hospital care codes [99231-99233] on the day of discharge.)

(For Observation Care Discharge, use 99217)

(For observation or inpatient hospital care including the admission and discharge of the patient on the same date, see 99234-99236)

(For Nursing Facility Care Discharge, see 99315, 99316)

(For discharge services provided to newborns admitted and discharged on the same date, use 99463)

Consultations

A consultation is a type of evaluation and management service provided at the request of another physician or appropriate source to either recommend care for a specific condition or problem or to determine whether to accept responsibility for ongoing management of the patient's entire care or for the care of a specific condition or problem.

A physician consultant may initiate diagnostic and/or therapeutic services at the same or subsequent visit.

A "consultation" initiated by a patient and/or family, and not requested by a physician or other appropriate source (eg, physician assistant, nurse practitioner, doctor of chiropractic, physical therapist, occupational therapist, speech-language pathologist, psychologist, social worker, lawyer, or insurance company), is not reported using the consultation codes but may be reported using the office visit, home service, or domiciliary/rest home care codes as appropriate.

The written or verbal request for consult may be made by a physician or other appropriate source and documented in the patient's medical record by either the consulting or requesting physician or appropriate source. The consultant's opinion and any services that were ordered or performed must also be documented in the patient's medical record and communicated by written report to the requesting physician or other appropriate source.

If a consultation is mandated (eg, by a third-party payer) modifier 32 should also be reported.

Any specifically identifiable procedure (ie, identified with a specific CPT code) performed on or subsequent to the date of the initial consultation should be reported separately.

If subsequent to the completion of a consultation the consultant assumes responsibility for management of a portion or all of the patient's condition(s), the appropriate

Evaluation and Management services code for the site of service should be reported. In the hospital or nursing facility setting, the consultant should use the appropriate inpatient consultation code for the initial encounter and then subsequent hospital or nursing facility care codes. In the office setting, the consultant should use the appropriate office or other outpatient consultation codes and then the established patient office or other outpatient services codes.

To report services provided to a patient who is admitted to a hospital or nursing facility in the course of an encounter in the office or other ambulatory facility, see the notes for Initial Hospital Inpatient Care (page 23 [of the *CPT 2021* codebook]) or Initial Nursing Facility Care (page 33 [of the *CPT 2021* codebook]).

For definitions of key components and commonly used terms, please see **Evaluation and Management Services Guidelines.**

Office or Other Outpatient Consultations

New or Established Patient

The following codes are used to report consultations provided in the office or in an outpatient or other ambulatory facility, including hospital observation services, home services, domiciliary, rest home, or emergency department (see the preceding consultation definition above). Follow-up visits in the consultant's office or other outpatient facility that are initiated by the consultant or patient are reported using the appropriate codes for established patients, office visits (99211-99215), domiciliary, rest home (99334-99337), or home (99347-99350). If an additional request for an opinion or advice regarding the same or a new problem is received from another physician or other appropriate source and documented in the medical record, the office consultation codes may be used again. Services that constitute transfer of care (ie, are provided for the management of the patient's entire care or for the care of a specific condition or problem) are reported with the appropriate new or established patient codes for office or other outpatient visits, domiciliary, rest home services, or home services.

Coding Tip

Definition of Transfer of Care

Transfer of care is the process whereby a physician or other qualified health care professional who is providing management for some or all of a patient's problems relinquishes this responsibility to another physician or other qualified health care professional who explicitly agrees to accept this responsibility and who, from the initial encounter, is not providing consultative services. The physician or other qualified health care professional transferring care is then no longer providing care for these problems though he or she may continue providing care for other conditions when appropriate. Consultation codes should not be reported by the physician or other qualified health care professional who has agreed to accept transfer of care before an initial evaluation but are appropriate to report if the decision to accept transfer of care cannot be made until after the initial consultation evaluation, regardless of site of service.

CPT Coding Guidelines, Evaluation and Management, Guidelines Common to All E/M Services, Concurrent Care and Transfer of Care

★ 99241 **Office consultation** for a new or established patient, which requires these 3 key components:

- **A problem focused history;**
- **A problem focused examination; and**
- **Straightforward medical decision making.**

Counseling and/or coordination of care with other physicians, other qualified health care professionals, or agencies are provided consistent with the nature of the problem(s) and the patient's and/or family's needs.

Usually, the presenting problem(s) are self limited or minor. Typically, 15 minutes are spent face-to-face with the patient and/or family.

➲ *CPT Changes: An Insider's View* 2013, 2017

➲ *CPT Assistant* Winter 91:11, Spring 92:4, 23-24, Summer 92:12, Spring 93:4, Spring 95:1, Oct 97:1, Sep 98:5, Jun 99:10, Apr 00:10, Aug 01:3, Jan 02:2, Jul 02:2, Sep 02:11, May 05:1, Dec 05:10, Jan 06:46, May 06:1, 16, Jun 06:1, Sep 06:8, Jan 07:28, Apr 07:11, Jul 07:1, May 08:13, Nov 08:10, Aug 09:9, Jan 10:3, Jul 10:4, Jun 11:3, Apr 12:10, Jan 13:9, Jun 13:3, Aug 14:3, Sep 14:13, Nov 14:14, Jan 15:12, Dec 15:18, Sep 16:6, Apr 18:10

➲ *Clinical Examples in Radiology* Summer 09:3

★ 99242 **Office consultation** for a new or established patient, which requires these 3 key components:

- **An expanded problem focused history;**
- **An expanded problem focused examination; and**
- **Straightforward medical decision making.**

Counseling and/or coordination of care with other physicians, other qualified health care professionals, or agencies are provided consistent with the nature of the problem(s) and the patient's and/or family's needs.

Usually, the presenting problem(s) are of low severity. Typically, 30 minutes are spent face-to-face with the patient and/or family.

➲ *CPT Changes: An Insider's View* 2000, 2013, 2017

➲ *CPT Assistant* Winter 91:11, Spring 92:4, 23-24, Summer 92:12, Spring 93:2, 34, Spring 95:1, Oct 97:1, Sep 98:5, Aug 01:3, Jan 02:2, Jul 02:2, Sep 02:11, Dec 05:10, May 06:1, 16, Jun 06:1, Sep 06:8, Apr 07:11, Jul 07:1, Jan 10:3, Jun 11:3, Jan 13:9, Jun 13:3, Sep 14:13, Jan 15:12, Sep 16:6, Apr 18:10

➲ *Clinical Examples in Radiology* Summer 09:3

★ 99243 **Office consultation** for a new or established patient, which requires these 3 key components:

- **A detailed history;**
- **A detailed examination; and**
- **Medical decision making of low complexity.**

Counseling and/or coordination of care with other physicians, other qualified health care professionals, or agencies are provided consistent with the nature of the problem(s) and the patient's and/or family's needs.

Usually, the presenting problem(s) are of moderate severity. Typically, 40 minutes are spent face-to-face with the patient and/or family.

➲ *CPT Changes: An Insider's View* 2013, 2017

➲ *CPT Assistant* Winter 91:11, Spring 92:4, 23-24, Summer 92:12, Spring 93:2, 34, Spring 95:1, Oct 97:1, Sep 98:5, Aug 01:3, Jan 02:2, Jul 02:2, Sep 02:11, Oct 03:5, Dec 05:10, May 06:1, 16, Jun 06:1, Sep 06:8, Apr 07:11, Jul 07:1, Jan 10:3, Jun 11:3, Jan 13:9, Jun 13:3, Sep 14:13, Jan 15:12, Sep 16:6, Apr 18:10

➲ *Clinical Examples in Radiology* Summer 09:3

★ **99244** **Office consultation** for a new or established patient, which requires these 3 key components:

- **A comprehensive history;**
- **A comprehensive examination; and**
- **Medical decision making of moderate complexity.**

Counseling and/or coordination of care with other physicians, other qualified health care professionals, or agencies are provided consistent with the nature of the problem(s) and the patient's and/or family's needs.

Usually, the presenting problem(s) are of moderate to high severity. Typically, 60 minutes are spent face-to-face with the patient and/or family.

➲ *CPT Changes: An Insider's View* 2013, 2017

➲ *CPT Assistant* Winter 91:11, Spring 92:3, 23-24, Summer 92:12, Spring 93:2, 34, Spring 95:1, Oct 97:1, Sep 98:5, Aug 01:3, Jan 02:2, Jul 02:2, Sep 02:11, Oct 03:5, Dec 05:10, May 06:1, 16, Jun 06:1, Sep 06:8, Apr 07:11, Jul 07:1, Jan 10:3, Jun 11:3, Jan 13:9, Jun 13:3, Aug 13:12, Sep 14:13, Jan 15:12, Sep 16:6, Apr 18:10

➲ *Clinical Examples in Radiology* Summer 09:2, 3

★ **99245** **Office consultation** for a new or established patient, which requires these 3 key components:

- **A comprehensive history;**
- **A comprehensive examination; and**
- **Medical decision making of high complexity.**

Counseling and/or coordination of care with other physicians, other qualified health care professionals, or agencies are provided consistent with the nature of the problem(s) and the patient's and/or family's needs.

Usually, the presenting problem(s) are of moderate to high severity. Typically, 80 minutes are spent face-to-face with the patient and/or family.

➲ *CPT Changes: An Insider's View* 2013, 2017

➲ *CPT Assistant* Winter 91:11, Spring 92:4, 23-24, Summer 92:12, Spring 93:2, 34, Spring 95:1, Oct 97:1, Sep 98:5, Aug 01:2, Jan 02:2, Jul 02:2, Sep 02:11, Dec 05:10, May 06:1, 16, Jun 06:1, Sep 06:8, Apr 07:11, Jul 07:1, Jan 10:3, Jul 10:4, Jun 11:3, Apr 12:10, Jan 13:9, Jun 13:3, Aug 14:3, Sep 14:13, Jan 15:12, Sep 16:6, Apr 18:10

➲ *Clinical Examples in Radiology* Summer 09:3

Inpatient Consultations

New or Established Patient

The following codes are used to report physician or other qualified health care professional consultations provided to hospital inpatients, residents of nursing facilities, or patients in a partial hospital setting. Only one consultation should be reported by a consultant per admission. Subsequent services during the same admission are reported using subsequent hospital care codes (99231-99233) or subsequent nursing facility care codes (99307-99310), including services to complete the initial consultation, monitor progress, revise recommendations, or address a new problem. Use subsequent hospital care codes (99231-99233) or subsequent nursing facility care codes (99307-99310) to report transfer of care services (see page 8 [of the *CPT 2021* codebook], Concurrent Care and Transfer of Care definitions).

When an inpatient consultation is performed on a date that a patient is admitted to a hospital or nursing facility, all evaluation and management services provided by the consultant related to the admission are reported with the inpatient consultation service code (99251-99255). If a patient is admitted after an outpatient consultation (office, emergency department, etc), and the patient is not seen on the unit on the date of admission, only report the outpatient consultation code (99241-99245). If the patient is seen by the consultant on the unit on the date of admission, report all evaluation and management services provided by the consultant related to the admission with either the inpatient consultation code (99251-99255) or with the initial inpatient admission service code (99221-99223). Do not report both an outpatient consultation (99241-99245) and inpatient consultation (99251-99255) for services related to the same inpatient stay. When transfer of care services are provided on a date subsequent to the outpatient consultation, use the subsequent hospital care codes (99231-99233) or subsequent nursing facility care codes (99307-99310).

★ **99251** **Inpatient consultation** for a new or established patient, which requires these 3 key components:

- **A problem focused history;**
- **A problem focused examination; and**
- **Straightforward medical decision making.**

Counseling and/or coordination of care with other physicians, other qualified health care professionals, or agencies are provided consistent with the nature of the problem(s) and the patient's and/or family's needs.

Usually, the presenting problem(s) are self limited or minor. Typically, 20 minutes are spent at the bedside and on the patient's hospital floor or unit.

➲ *CPT Changes: An Insider's View* 2007, 2013, 2017

➲ *CPT Assistant* Winter 91:11, Spring 92:16, 23-24, Summer 92:12, Spring 93:34, Spring 95:1, Oct 97:1, Sep 98:5, Aug 01:3, Sep 02:11, May 05:1, May 06:1, 16, Jun 06:1, Jul 06:19, Jul 07:1, Jan 10:3, Jan 13:9, Jun 13:3

➲ *Clinical Examples in Radiology* Summer 09:3

★ **99252** **Inpatient consultation** for a new or established patient, which requires these 3 key components:

- **An expanded problem focused history;**
- **An expanded problem focused examination; and**
- **Straightforward medical decision making.**

Counseling and/or coordination of care with other physicians, other qualified health care professionals, or agencies are provided consistent with the nature of the problem(s) and the patient's and/or family's needs.

Usually, the presenting problem(s) are of low severity. Typically, 40 minutes are spent at the bedside and on the patient's hospital floor or unit.

➲ *CPT Changes: An Insider's View* 2007, 2013, 2017

➲ *CPT Assistant* Winter 91:11, Spring 92:16, 23-24, Summer 92:12, Summer 93:34, Spring 95:1, Oct 97:1, Sep 98:5, Aug 01:4, Sep 02:11, May 06:1, 16, Jun 06:1, Jul 06:19, Jul 07:1, Jan 10:3, Jan 13:9, Jun 13:3

➲ *Clinical Examples in Radiology* Summer 09:3

★ **99253** **Inpatient consultation** for a new or established patient, which requires these 3 key components:

- **A detailed history;**
- **A detailed examination; and**
- **Medical decision making of low complexity.**

Counseling and/or coordination of care with other physicians, other qualified health care professionals, or agencies are provided consistent with the nature of the problem(s) and the patient's and/or family's needs.

Usually, the presenting problem(s) are of moderate severity. Typically, 55 minutes are spent at the bedside and on the patient's hospital floor or unit.

➲ *CPT Changes: An Insider's View* 2007, 2013, 2017

➲ *CPT Assistant* Winter 91:11, Spring 92:16, 23-24, Summer 92:12, Summer 93:34, Spring 95:1, Oct 97:1, Sep 98:5, Aug 01:4, Sep 02:11, May 06:1, 16, Jun 06:1, Jul 06:19, Jul 07:1, Jan 10:3, Jan 13:9, Jun 13:3

➲ *Clinical Examples in Radiology* Summer 09:3

★ **99254** **Inpatient consultation** for a new or established patient, which requires these 3 key components:

- **A comprehensive history;**
- **A comprehensive examination; and**
- **Medical decision making of moderate complexity.**

Counseling and/or coordination of care with other physicians, other qualified health care professionals, or agencies are provided consistent with the nature of the problem(s) and the patient's and/or family's needs.

Usually, the presenting problem(s) are of moderate to high severity. Typically, 80 minutes are spent at the bedside and on the patient's hospital floor or unit.

➲ *CPT Changes: An Insider's View* 2007, 2013, 2017

➲ *CPT Assistant* Winter 91:11, Spring 92:16, 23-24, Summer 92:12, Summer 93:34, Spring 95:1, Oct 97:1, Sep 98:5, Aug 01:4, Sep 02:11, May 06:1, 16, Jun 06:1, Jul 06:19, Jul 07:1, Jan 10:3, Jan 13:9, Jun 13:3

➲ *Clinical Examples in Radiology* Summer 09:3

★ **99255** **Inpatient consultation** for a new or established patient, which requires these 3 key components:

- **A comprehensive history;**
- **A comprehensive examination; and**
- **Medical decision making of high complexity.**

Counseling and/or coordination of care with other physicians, other qualified health care professionals, or agencies are provided consistent with the nature of the problem(s) and the patient's and/or family's needs.

Usually, the presenting problem(s) are of moderate to high severity. Typically, 110 minutes are spent at the bedside and on the patient's hospital floor or unit.

➲ *CPT Changes: An Insider's View* 2007, 2013, 2017

➲ *CPT Assistant* Winter 91:11, Spring 92:16, 23-24, Summer 92:12, Summer 93:34, Spring 95:1, Oct 97:1, Sep 98:5, Aug 01:4, Sep 02:11, May 06:1, 16, Jun 06:1, Jul 06:19, Jul 07:1, Jan 10:3, Jan 13:9, Jun 13:3, Nov 14:14

➲ *Clinical Examples in Radiology* Summer 09:3

Emergency Department Services

New or Established Patient

The following codes are used to report evaluation and management services provided in the emergency department. No distinction is made between new and established patients in the emergency department.

An emergency department is defined as an organized hospital-based facility for the provision of unscheduled episodic services to patients who present for immediate medical attention. The facility must be available 24 hours a day.

For critical care services provided in the emergency department, see Critical Care notes and 99291, 99292.

For evaluation and management services provided to a patient in an observation area of a hospital, see 99217-99220.

For observation or inpatient care services (including admission and discharge services), see 99234-99236.

Coding Tip

Time as a Factor in the Emergency Department Setting

Time is **not** a descriptive component for the emergency department levels of E/M services because emergency department services are typically provided on a variable intensity basis, often involving multiple encounters with several patients over an extended period of time. Therefore, it is often difficult for physicians to provide accurate estimates of the time spent face-to-face with the patient.

CPT Coding Guidelines, Evaluation and Management, Guidelines Common to All E/M Services, Time

---

99281 **Emergency department visit** for the evaluation and management of a patient, which requires these 3 key components:

- **A problem focused history;**
- **A problem focused examination; and**
- **Straightforward medical decision making.**

Counseling and/or coordination of care with other physicians, other qualified health care professionals, or agencies are provided consistent with the nature of the problem(s) and the patient's and/or family's needs.

Usually, the presenting problem(s) are self limited or minor.

➲ *CPT Changes: An Insider's View* 2013

➲ *CPT Assistant* Winter 91:11, Spring 92:24, Summer 92:18, Spring 93:34, Spring 95:1, Feb 96:3, Sep 98:5, Jan 00:11, Feb 00:11, Sep 00:3, Apr 02:14, Jul 02:2, Nov 05:10, Feb 06:14, Dec 06:14, Dec 07:13, Jan 13:9, Jun 13:3, Nov 14:14, Jan 15:12, Jul 19:10

99282 **Emergency department visit** for the evaluation and management of a patient, which requires these 3 key components:

- **An expanded problem focused history;**
- **An expanded problem focused examination; and**
- **Medical decision making of low complexity.**

Counseling and/or coordination of care with other physicians, other qualified health care professionals, or agencies are provided consistent with the nature of the problem(s) and the patient's and/or family's needs.

Usually, the presenting problem(s) are of low to moderate severity.

➲ *CPT Changes: An Insider's View* 2013

➲ *CPT Assistant* Winter 91:11, Spring 92:24, Summer 92:18, Spring 93:34, Spring 95:1, Summer 95:1, Feb 96:3, Sep 98:5, Jan 00:11, Feb 00:11, Sep 00:3, Apr 02:14, Jul 02:2, Nov 05:10, Feb 06:14, Dec 06:14, Dec 07:13, Jan 13:9, Jun 13:3, Jan 15:12, Jul 19:10

99283 **Emergency department visit** for the evaluation and management of a patient, which requires these 3 key components:

- **An expanded problem focused history;**
- **An expanded problem focused examination; and**
- **Medical decision making of moderate complexity.**

Counseling and/or coordination of care with other physicians, other qualified health care professionals, or agencies are provided consistent with the nature of the problem(s) and the patient's and/or family's needs.

Usually, the presenting problem(s) are of moderate severity.

➲ *CPT Changes: An Insider's View* 2013

➲ *CPT Assistant* Winter 91:11, Spring 92:24, Summer 92:18, Spring 93:34, Spring 95:1, Summer 95:1, Feb 96:3, Sep 98:5, Jan 00:11, Feb 00:11, Sep 00:3, Apr 02:14, Jul 02:2, Nov 05:10, Feb 06:14, Dec 06:14, Dec 07:13, Jan 13:9, Jun 13:3, Jan 15:12, Jul 19:10

99284 **Emergency department visit** for the evaluation and management of a patient, which requires these 3 key components:

- **A detailed history;**
- **A detailed examination; and**
- **Medical decision making of moderate complexity.**

Counseling and/or coordination of care with other physicians, other qualified health care professionals, or agencies are provided consistent with the nature of the problem(s) and the patient's and/or family's needs.

Usually, the presenting problem(s) are of high severity, and require urgent evaluation by the physician, or other qualified health care professionals but do not pose an immediate significant threat to life or physiologic function.

➲ *CPT Changes: An Insider's View* 2013

➲ *CPT Assistant* Winter 91:11, Spring 92:24, Summer 92:18, Spring 93:34, Spring 95:1, Summer 95:1, Feb 96:3, Sep 98:5, Jan 00:11, Feb 00:11, Sep 00:3, Apr 02:14, Jul 02:2, Nov 05:10, Feb 06:14, Dec 06:14, Dec 07:13, Jan 13:9, Jun 13:3, Jan 15:12, Jul 19:10

99285 **Emergency department visit** for the evaluation and management of a patient, which requires these 3 key components within the constraints imposed by the urgency of the patient's clinical condition and/or mental status:

- **A comprehensive history;**
- **A comprehensive examination; and**
- **Medical decision making of high complexity.**

Counseling and/or coordination of care with other physicians, other qualified health care professionals, or agencies are provided consistent with the nature of the problem(s) and the patient's and/or family's needs.

Usually, the presenting problem(s) are of high severity and pose an immediate significant threat to life or physiologic function.

➲ *CPT Changes: An Insider's View* 2000, 2013

➲ *CPT Assistant* Winter 91:11, Spring 92:24, Summer 92:18, Spring 93:34, Spring 95:1, Summer 95:1, Feb 96:3, Aug 98:8, Sep 98:5, Nov 99:23, Jan 00:11, Feb 00:11, Sep 00:3, Apr 02:14, Jul 02:2, Sep 02:11, Mar 05:11, Nov 05:10, Feb 06:14, Dec 06:14, Dec 07:13, Jan 13:9, Jun 13:3, Nov 14:14, Jan 15:12, Jul 19:10, Jan 20:12

Coding Tip

Emergency Department Classification of New vs Established Patient

No distinction is made between new and established patients in the emergency department. E/M services in the emergency department category may be reported for any new or established patient who presents for treatment in the emergency department.

CPT Coding Guidelines, Evaluation and Management, Guidelines Common to All E/M Services, New and Established Patient

Other Emergency Services

In directed emergency care, advanced life support, the physician or other qualified health care professional is located in a hospital emergency or critical care department, and is in two-way voice communication with ambulance or rescue personnel outside the hospital. Direction of the performance of necessary medical procedures includes but is not limited to: telemetry of cardiac rhythm; cardiac and/or pulmonary resuscitation; endotracheal or esophageal obturator airway intubation; administration of intravenous fluids and/or administration of intramuscular, intratracheal or subcutaneous drugs; and/or electrical conversion of arrhythmia.

99288 **Physician or other qualified health care professional direction of** emergency medical systems (EMS) emergency care, advanced life support

➲ *CPT Changes: An Insider's View* 2013

➲ *CPT Assistant* Summer 92:18, May 05:1, Nov 07:5, May 13:6

Critical Care Services

Critical care is the direct delivery by a physician(s) or other qualified health care professional of medical care for a critically ill or critically injured patient. A critical illness or injury acutely impairs one or more vital organ systems such that there is a high probability of imminent or life threatening deterioration in the patient's condition. Critical care involves high complexity decision making to assess, manipulate, and support vital system function(s) to treat single or multiple vital organ system failure and/or to prevent further life threatening deterioration of the patient's condition. Examples of vital organ system failure include, but are not limited to: central nervous system failure, circulatory failure, shock, renal, hepatic, metabolic, and/or respiratory failure. Although critical care typically requires interpretation of multiple physiologic parameters and/or application of advanced technology(s), critical care may be provided in life threatening situations when these elements are not present. Critical care may be provided on multiple days, even if no changes are made in the treatment rendered to the patient, provided that the patient's condition continues to require the level of attention described above.

Providing medical care to a critically ill, injured, or post-operative patient qualifies as a critical care service only if both the illness or injury and the treatment being provided meet the above requirements. Critical care is usually, but not always, given in a critical care area, such as the coronary care unit, intensive care unit, pediatric intensive care unit, respiratory care unit, or the emergency care facility.

Inpatient critical care services provided to infants 29 days through 71 months of age are reported with pediatric critical care codes 99471-99476. The pediatric critical care codes are reported as long as the infant/young child qualifies for critical care services during the hospital stay through 71 months of age. Inpatient critical care services provided to neonates (28 days of age or younger) are reported with the neonatal critical care codes 99468 and 99469. The neonatal critical care codes are reported as long as the neonate qualifies for critical care services during the hospital stay through the 28th postnatal day. The reporting of the pediatric and neonatal critical care services is not based on time or the type of unit (eg, pediatric or neonatal critical care unit) and it is not dependent upon the type of physician or other qualified health care professional delivering the care. To report critical care services provided in the outpatient setting (eg, emergency department or office), for neonates and pediatric patients up through 71 months of age, see the critical care codes 99291, 99292. If the same individual provides critical care services for a neonatal or pediatric patient in both the outpatient and inpatient settings on the same day, report only the appropriate neonatal or pediatric critical care code 99468-99472 for all critical care services provided on that day. Also report 99291-99292 for neonatal or pediatric critical care services provided by the individual providing critical care at one facility but transferring the patient to another facility. Critical care services provided by a second individual of a different specialty not reporting a per day neonatal or pediatric critical care code can be reported with codes 99291, 99292. For additional instructions on reporting these services, see the Neonatal and Pediatric Critical Care section and codes 99468-99476.

Services for a patient who is not critically ill but happens to be in a critical care unit are reported using other appropriate E/M codes.

Critical care and other E/M services may be provided to the same patient on the same date by the same individual.

For reporting by professionals, the following services are included in critical care when performed during the critical period by the physician(s) providing critical care: the interpretation of cardiac output measurements (93561, 93562), chest X rays (71045, 71046), pulse oximetry (94760, 94761, 94762), blood gases, and collection and interpretation of physiologic data (eg, ECGs, blood pressures, hematologic data); gastric intubation (43752, 43753); temporary transcutaneous pacing (92953); ventilatory management (94002-94004, 94660, 94662); and vascular access procedures (36000, 36410, 36415, 36591, 36600). Any services performed that are not included in this listing should be reported separately. Facilities may report the above services separately.

Codes 99291, 99292 should be reported for the attendance during the transport of critically ill or critically injured patients older than 24 months of age to or from a facility or hospital. For transport services of critically ill or critically injured pediatric patients 24 months of age or younger, see 99466, 99467.

Codes 99291, 99292 are used to report the total duration of time spent in provision of critical care services to a critically ill or critically injured patient, even if the time spent providing care on that date is not continuous. For any given period of time spent providing critical care services, the individual must devote his or her full attention to the patient and, therefore, cannot provide services to any other patient during the same period of time.

Time spent with the individual patient should be recorded in the patient's record. The time that can be reported as critical care is the time spent engaged in work directly related to the individual patient's care whether that time was spent at the immediate bedside or elsewhere on the floor or unit. For example, time spent on the unit or at the nursing station on the floor reviewing test results or imaging studies, discussing the critically ill patient's care with other medical staff or documenting critical care services in the medical record would be reported as critical care, even though it does not occur at the bedside. Also, when the patient is unable or lacks capacity to participate in discussions, time spent on the floor or unit with family members or surrogate decision makers obtaining a medical history, reviewing the patient's condition or prognosis, or discussing treatment or limitation(s) of treatment may be reported as critical care, provided that the conversation bears directly on the management of the patient.

Time spent in activities that occur outside of the unit or off the floor (eg, telephone calls whether taken at home, in the office, or elsewhere in the hospital) may not be reported as critical care since the individual is not immediately available to the patient. Time spent in activities that do not directly contribute to the treatment of the patient may not be reported as critical care, even if they are performed in the critical care unit (eg, participation in administrative meetings or telephone calls to discuss other patients). Time spent performing separately reportable procedures or services should not be included in the time reported as critical care time.

Code 99291 is used to report the first 30-74 minutes of critical care on a given date. It should be used only once per date even if the time spent by the individual is not continuous on that date. Critical care of less than 30 minutes total duration on a given date should be reported with the appropriate E/M code.

Code 99292 is used to report additional block(s) of time, of up to 30 minutes each beyond the first 74 minutes. (See the following table.)

The following examples illustrate the correct reporting of critical care services:

Total Duration of Critical Care Codes

less than 30 minutes	appropriate E/M codes
30-74 minutes (30 minutes - 1 hr. 14 min.)	99291 X 1
75-104 minutes (1 hr. 15 min. - 1 hr. 44 min.)	99291 X 1 AND 99292 X 1
105-134 minutes (1 hr. 45 min. - 2 hr. 14 min.)	99291 X 1 AND 99292 X 2
135-164 minutes (2 hr. 15 min. - 2 hr. 44 min.)	99291 X 1 AND 99292 X 3
165-194 minutes (2 hr. 45 min. - 3 hr. 14 min.)	99291 X 1 AND 99292 X 4
195 minutes or longer (3 hr. 15 min. - etc.)	99291 and 99292 as appropriate (see illustrated reporting examples above)

99291 **Critical care, evaluation and management** of the critically ill or critically injured patient; first 30-74 minutes

➲ *CPT Assistant* Summer 92:18, Summer 93:1, Summer 95:1, Jan 96:7, Apr 97:3, Dec 98:6, Nov 99:3, Apr 00:6, Sep 00:1, Dec 00:15, Jul 02:2, Feb 03:15, Oct 03:2, Aug 04:7, 10, Oct 04:14, May 05:1, Jul 05:15, Nov 05:10, Jul 06:4, Dec 06:13, Nov 07:5, Jan 09:5, Mar 09:3, Jul 09:10, Aug 11:10, Sep 11:3, Jul 12:13, Feb 13:17, May 13:6, May 14:4, Aug 14:5, Oct 14:14, Feb 15:10, May 16:3, Aug 16:9, Oct 16:8, Jun 18:9, Dec 18:8, Jul 19:10, Aug 19:8, Dec 19:14, Jan 20:12, Feb 20:7

+ 99292 each additional 30 minutes (List separately in addition to code for primary service)

➲ *CPT Assistant* Summer 92:18, Summer 93:1, Summer 95:1, Jan 96:7, Apr 97:3, Dec 98:6, Nov 99:3, Apr 00:6, Sep 00:1, Dec 00:15, Feb 03:15, Oct 03:2, Aug 04:10, Oct 04:14, Jul 05:15, Nov 05:10, Jul 06:4, Dec 06:13, Nov 07:5, Jan 09:5, Mar 09:3, Aug 11:10, Sep 11:3, Feb 13:17, May 13:6, May 14:4, Aug 14:5, Oct 14:14, Feb 15:10, May 16:3, Aug 16:9, Jun 18:9, Dec 18:8, Jul 19:10, Aug 19:8, Dec 19:14, Feb 20:7

(Use 99292 in conjunction with 99291)

Coding Tip

Services Included in Critical Care Services

For reporting by professionals, the following services are included in critical care when performed during the critical period by the physician(s) providing critical care: the interpretation of cardiac output measurements (93561, 93562), chest X rays (71045, 71046), pulse oximetry (94760, 94761, 94762), blood gases, and collection and interpretation of physiologic data (eg, ECGs, blood pressures, hematologic data); gastric intubation (43752, 43753); temporary transcutaneous pacing (92953); ventilatory management (94002-94004, 94660, 94662); and vascular access procedures (36000, 36410, 36415, 36591, 36600). Any services performed that are not listed above should be reported separately. Facilities may report the above services separately

CPT Coding Guideline, Critical Care

Nursing Facility Services

The following codes are used to report evaluation and management services to patients in nursing facilities (formerly called skilled nursing facilities [SNFs], intermediate care facilities [ICFs], or long-term care facilities [LTCFs]).

These codes should also be used to report evaluation and management services provided to a patient in a psychiatric residential treatment center (a facility or a distinct part of a facility for psychiatric care, which provides a 24-hour therapeutically planned and professionally staffed group living and learning environment). If procedures such as medical psychotherapy are provided in addition to evaluation and management services, these should be reported in addition to the evaluation and management services provided.

Nursing facilities that provide convalescent, rehabilitative, or long term care are required to conduct comprehensive, accurate, standardized, and reproducible assessments of each resident's functional capacity using a Resident Assessment Instrument (RAI). All RAIs include the Minimum Data Set (MDS), Resident Assessment Protocols (RAPs), and utilization guidelines. The MDS is the primary screening and assessment tool; the RAPs trigger the identification of potential problems and provide guidelines for follow-up assessments.

Physicians have a central role in assuring that all residents receive thorough assessments and that medical plans of care are instituted or revised to enhance or maintain the residents' physical and psychosocial functioning. This role includes providing input in the development of the MDS and a multi-disciplinary plan of care, as required by regulations pertaining to the care of nursing facility residents.

Two major subcategories of nursing facility services are recognized: Initial Nursing Facility Care and Subsequent Nursing Facility Care. Both subcategories apply to new or established patients.

For definitions of key components and commonly used terms, please see **Evaluation and Management Services Guidelines.**

(For care plan oversight services provided to nursing facility residents, see 99379-99380)

Initial Nursing Facility Care

New or Established Patient

When the patient is admitted to the nursing facility in the course of an encounter in another site of service (eg, hospital emergency department, office), all evaluation and management services provided by that physician in conjunction with that admission are considered part of the initial nursing facility care when performed on the same date as the admission or readmission. The nursing facility care level of service reported by the admitting physician should include the services related to the admission he/she provided in the other sites of service as well as in the nursing facility setting.

Hospital discharge or observation discharge services performed on the same date of nursing facility admission or readmission may be reported separately. For a patient discharged from inpatient status on the same date of nursing facility admission or readmission, the hospital discharge services should be reported with codes 99238, 99239 as appropriate. For a patient discharged from observation status on the same date of nursing facility admission or readmission, the observation care discharge services should be reported with code 99217. For a patient admitted and discharged from observation or inpatient status on the same date, see codes 99234-99236.

(For nursing facility care discharge, see 99315, 99316)

Coding Tip

The Significance of Time as a Factor in Selection of an Evaluation and Management Code from This Section

The inclusion of time as an explicit factor beginning in CPT 1992 was done to assist in selecting the most appropriate level of E/M services included in codes in this section. Beginning with CPT 2021, except for 99211, time alone may be used to select the appropriate code level for the office or other outpatient E/M services codes (99202, 99203, 99204, 99205, 99212, 99213, 99214, 99215). Different categories of services use time differently. It is important to review the instructions for each category.

Unit/floor time (hospital observation services [99218, 99219, 99220, 99224, 99225, 99226, 99234, 99235, 99236], hospital inpatient services [99221, 99222, 99223, 99231, 99232, 99233], inpatient consultations [99251, 99252, 99253, 99254, 99255], nursing facility services [99304, 99305, 99306, 99307, 99308, 99309, 99310, 99315, 99316, 99318]):

For coding purposes, time for these services is defined as unit/floor time, which includes the time present on the patient's hospital unit and at the bedside rendering services for that patient. This includes the time to establish and/or review the patient's chart, examine the patient, write notes, and communicate with other professionals and the patient's family.

CPT Coding Guidelines, Evaluation and Management, Guidelines Common to All E/M Services, Time

---

99304 Initial nursing facility care, per day, for the evaluation and management of a patient, which requires these 3 key components:

- **A detailed or comprehensive history;**
- **A detailed or comprehensive examination; and**
- **Medical decision making that is straightforward or of low complexity.**

Counseling and/or coordination of care with other physicians, other qualified health care professionals, or agencies are provided consistent with the nature of the problem(s) and the patient's and/or family's needs.

Usually, the problem(s) requiring admission are of low severity. Typically, 25 minutes are spent at the bedside and on the patient's facility floor or unit.

➲ *CPT Changes: An Insider's View* 2006, 2008, 2010, 2013

➲ *CPT Assistant* Jul 10:4, Jan 11:3, Jun 11:3, Jan 12:3, Jul 12:12, Jan 13:9, Jun 13:3, Nov 14:14

99305 Initial nursing facility care, per day, for the evaluation and management of a patient, which requires these 3 key components:

- **A comprehensive history;**
- **A comprehensive examination; and**
- **Medical decision making of moderate complexity.**

Counseling and/or coordination of care with other physicians, other qualified health care professionals, or agencies are provided consistent with the nature of the problem(s) and the patient's and/or family's needs.

Usually, the problem(s) requiring admission are of moderate severity. Typically, 35 minutes are spent at the bedside and on the patient's facility floor or unit.

➲ *CPT Changes: An Insider's View* 2006, 2008, 2010, 2013

➲ *CPT Assistant* Jan 11:3, Jun 11:3, Jul 12:12, Jan 13:9, Jun 13:3

99306 Initial nursing facility care, per day, for the evaluation and management of a patient, which requires these 3 key components:

- **A comprehensive history;**
- **A comprehensive examination; and**
- **Medical decision making of high complexity.**

Counseling and/or coordination of care with other physicians, other qualified health care professionals, or agencies are provided consistent with the nature of the problem(s) and the patient's and/or family's needs.

Usually, the problem(s) requiring admission are of high severity. Typically, 45 minutes are spent at the bedside and on the patient's facility floor or unit.

CPT Changes: An Insider's View 2006, 2008, 2010, 2013

CPT Assistant Jan 11:3, Jun 11:3, Jan 12:3, Jul 12:12, Jan 13:9, Jun 13:3

Subsequent Nursing Facility Care

All levels of subsequent nursing facility care include reviewing the medical record and reviewing the results of diagnostic studies and changes in the patient's status (ie, changes in history, physical condition, and response to management) since the last assessment by the physician or other qualified health are professional.

★ **99307** Subsequent nursing facility care, per day, for the evaluation and management of a patient, which requires at least 2 of these 3 key components:

- **A problem focused interval history;**
- **A problem focused examination;**
- **Straightforward medical decision making.**

Counseling and/or coordination of care with other physicians, other qualified health care professionals, or agencies are provided consistent with the nature of the problem(s) and the patient's and/or family's needs.

Usually, the patient is stable, recovering, or improving. Typically, 10 minutes are spent at the bedside and on the patient's facility floor or unit.

CPT Changes: An Insider's View 2006, 2008, 2010, 2013, 2017

CPT Assistant May 06:1, 16, Jun 06:1, 19, Mar 07:9, Jul 07:1, Jul 09:3, 8, Jan 11:3, Jan 12:3, Jul 12:12, Jan 13:9, Jun 13:3

★ **99308** Subsequent nursing facility care, per day, for the evaluation and management of a patient, which requires at least 2 of these 3 key components:

- **An expanded problem focused interval history;**
- **An expanded problem focused examination;**
- **Medical decision making of low complexity.**

Counseling and/or coordination of care with other physicians, other qualified health care professionals, or agencies are provided consistent with the nature of the problem(s) and the patient's and/or family's needs.

Usually, the patient is responding inadequately to therapy or has developed a minor complication. Typically, 15 minutes are spent at the bedside and on the patient's facility floor or unit.

CPT Changes: An Insider's View 2006, 2008, 2010, 2013, 2017

CPT Assistant May 06:1, 16, Jun 06:1, 19, Mar 07:9, Jul 07:1, Jul 09:3, 8, Jan 11:3, Jul 12:12, Jan 13:9, Jun 13:3

99325 Domiciliary or rest home visit for the evaluation and management of a new patient, which requires these 3 key components:

- **An expanded problem focused history;**
- **An expanded problem focused examination; and**
- **Medical decision making of low complexity.**

Counseling and/or coordination of care with other physicians, other qualified health care professionals, or agencies are provided consistent with the nature of the problem(s) and the patient's and/or family's needs.

Usually, the presenting problem(s) are of moderate severity. Typically, 30 minutes are spent with the patient and/or family or caregiver.

➲ *CPT Changes: An Insider's View* 2006, 2013

➲ *CPT Assistant* Jan 06:1, Jun 06:1, Jul 09:8, Aug 09:5, Jan 11:3, Jan 13:9, Jun 13:3

99326 Domiciliary or rest home visit for the evaluation and management of a new patient, which requires these 3 key components:

- **A detailed history;**
- **A detailed examination; and**
- **Medical decision making of moderate complexity.**

Counseling and/or coordination of care with other physicians, other qualified health care professionals, or agencies are provided consistent with the nature of the problem(s) and the patient's and/or family's needs.

Usually, the presenting problem(s) are of moderate to high severity. Typically, 45 minutes are spent with the patient and/or family or caregiver.

➲ *CPT Changes: An Insider's View* 2006, 2013

➲ *CPT Assistant* Jan 06:1, Jun 06:1, Jul 09:8, Aug 09:5, Jan 11:3, Jan 13:9, Jun 13:3

99327 Domiciliary or rest home visit for the evaluation and management of a new patient, which requires these 3 key components:

- **A comprehensive history;**
- **A comprehensive examination; and**
- **Medical decision making of moderate complexity.**

Counseling and/or coordination of care with other physicians, other qualified health care professionals, or agencies are provided consistent with the nature of the problem(s) and the patient's and/or family's needs.

Usually, the presenting problem(s) are of high severity. Typically, 60 minutes are spent with the patient and/or family or caregiver.

➲ *CPT Changes: An Insider's View* 2006, 2013

➲ *CPT Assistant* Jan 06:1, Jun 06:1, Jul 09:8, Aug 09:5, Jan 11:3, Jan 13:9, Jun 13:3

99328 Domiciliary or rest home visit for the evaluation and management of a new patient, which requires these 3 key components:

- **A comprehensive history;**
- **A comprehensive examination; and**
- **Medical decision making of high complexity.**

Counseling and/or coordination of care with other physicians, other qualified health care professionals, or agencies are provided consistent with the nature of the problem(s) and the patient's and/or family's needs.

Usually, the patient is unstable or has developed a significant new problem requiring immediate physician attention. Typically, 75 minutes are spent with the patient and/or family or caregiver.

➲ *CPT Changes: An Insider's View* 2006, 2013

➲ *CPT Assistant* Jan 06:1, Jun 06:1, Jul 09:8, Aug 09:5, Jan 11:3, Jan 12:3, Jan 13:9, Jun 13:3

Established Patient

99334 Domiciliary or rest home visit for the evaluation and management of an established patient, which requires at least 2 of these 3 key components:

- **A problem focused interval history;**
- **A problem focused examination;**
- **Straightforward medical decision making.**

Counseling and/or coordination of care with other physicians, other qualified health care professionals, or agencies are provided consistent with the nature of the problem(s) and the patient's and/or family's needs.

Usually, the presenting problem(s) are self-limited or minor. Typically, 15 minutes are spent with the patient and/or family or caregiver.

➲ *CPT Changes: An Insider's View* 2006, 2013

➲ *CPT Assistant* Jan 06:1, Jun 06:1, Jul 07:1, Jul 09:8, Aug 09:5, Jan 11:3, Jan 12:3, Jan 13:9, Jun 13:3, Nov 13:3

99335 Domiciliary or rest home visit for the evaluation and management of an established patient, which requires at least 2 of these 3 key components:

- **An expanded problem focused interval history;**
- **An expanded problem focused examination;**
- **Medical decision making of low complexity.**

Counseling and/or coordination of care with other physicians, other qualified health care professionals, or agencies are provided consistent with the nature of the problem(s) and the patient's and/or family's needs.

Usually, the presenting problem(s) are of low to moderate severity. Typically, 25 minutes are spent with the patient and/or family or caregiver.

➲ *CPT Changes: An Insider's View* 2006, 2013

➲ *CPT Assistant* Jan 06:1, Jun 06:1, Jul 07:1, Jul 09:8, Aug 09:5, Jan 11:3, Jan 13:9, Jun 13:3

99336 Domiciliary or rest home visit for the evaluation and management of an established patient, which requires at least 2 of these 3 key components:

- **A detailed interval history;**
- **A detailed examination;**
- **Medical decision making of moderate complexity.**

Counseling and/or coordination of care with other physicians, other qualified health care professionals, or agencies are provided consistent with the nature of the problem(s) and the patient's and/or family's needs.

Usually, the presenting problem(s) are of moderate to high severity. Typically, 40 minutes are spent with the patient and/or family or caregiver.

➲ *CPT Changes: An Insider's View* 2006, 2013

➲ *CPT Assistant* Jan 06:1, Jun 06:1, Jul 07:1, Jul 09:8, Aug 09:5, Jan 11:3, Jan 13:9, Jun 13:3

99337 Domiciliary or rest home visit for the evaluation and management of an established patient, which requires at least 2 of these 3 key components:

- **A comprehensive interval history;**
- **A comprehensive examination;**
- **Medical decision making of moderate to high complexity.**

Counseling and/or coordination of care with other physicians, other qualified health care professionals, or agencies are provided consistent with the nature of the problem(s) and the patient's and/or family's needs.

Usually, the presenting problem(s) are of moderate to high severity. The patient may be unstable or may have developed a significant new problem requiring immediate physician attention. Typically, 60 minutes are spent with the patient and/or family or caregiver.

➲ *CPT Changes: An Insider's View* 2006, 2013

➲ *CPT Assistant* Jan 06:1, Jun 06:1, Jul 07:1, Jul 09:8, Aug 09:5, Jan 11:3, Jan 12:3, Apr 12:10, Jan 13:9, Jun 13:3, Nov 13:3, Oct 14:3, Nov 14:14

Domiciliary, Rest Home (eg, Assisted Living Facility), or Home Care Plan Oversight Services

(For instructions on the use of 99339, 99340, see introductory notes for 99374-99380)

(For care plan oversight services for patients under the care of a home health agency, hospice, or nursing facility, see 99374-99380)

(Do not report 99339, 99340 for time reported with 98966, 98967, 98968, 99421, 99422, 99423, 99441, 99442, 99443)

99339 Individual physician supervision of a patient (patient not present) in home, domiciliary or rest home (eg, assisted living facility) requiring complex and multidisciplinary care modalities involving regular physician development and/or revision of care plans, review of subsequent reports of patient status, review of related laboratory and other studies, communication (including telephone calls) for purposes of assessment or care decisions with health care professional(s), family member(s), surrogate decision maker(s) (eg, legal guardian) and/or key caregiver(s) involved in patient's care, integration of new information into the medical treatment plan and/or adjustment of medical therapy, within a calendar month; 15-29 minutes

➲ *CPT Changes: An Insider's View* 2006

➲ *CPT Assistant* Jan 06:1, Dec 06:4, Mar 07:11, Sep 08:3, Jul 09:5, 10, Jan 12:3, Apr 13:3, Jun 13:3, Sep 13:15, Nov 13:3, Oct 14:3

99340 30 minutes or more

➲ *CPT Changes: An Insider's View* 2006

➲ *CPT Assistant* Jan 06:1, Dec 06:4, Mar 07:11, Sep 08:3, Jul 09:5, 10, Jan 12:3, Apr 13:3, Jun 13:3, Sep 13:15, Nov 13:3, Oct 14:3

(Do not report 99339, 99340 for patients under the care of a home health agency, enrolled in a hospice program, or for nursing facility residents)

(Do not report 99339, 99340 during the same month with 99487-99489)

Home Services

The following codes are used to report evaluation and management services provided in a home. Home may be defined as a private residence, temporary lodging, or short term accommodation (eg, hotel, campground, hostel, or cruise ship).

For definitions of key components and commonly used terms, please see **Evaluation and Management Services Guidelines.**

(For care plan oversight services provided to a patient in the home under the care of a home health agency, see 99374, 99375, and for hospice agency, see 99377, 99378. For care plan oversight provided to a patient under hospice or home health agency care, see 99339, 99340)

New Patient

99341 **Home visit** for the evaluation and management of a new patient, which requires these 3 key components:

- **A problem focused history;**
- **A problem focused examination; and**
- **Straightforward medical decision making.**

Counseling and/or coordination of care with other physicians, other qualified health care professionals, or agencies are provided consistent with the nature of the problem(s) and the patient's and/or family's needs.

Usually, the presenting problem(s) are of low severity. Typically, 20 minutes are spent face-to-face with the patient and/or family.

➲ *CPT Changes: An Insider's View* 2013

➲ *CPT Assistant* Winter 91:11, Spring 92:24, Summer 92:12, Spring 93:34, Spring 95:1, Jun 97:6, Nov 97:6-8, Oct 98:6, Oct 03:7, May 05:1, Jan 06:1, Jul 09:8, Aug 09:5, Jan 11:3, Jan 12:3, Apr 12:10, Jan 13:9, Jun 13:3, Oct 14:3, Nov 14:14

99342 **Home visit** for the evaluation and management of a new patient, which requires these 3 key components:

- **An expanded problem focused history;**
- **An expanded problem focused examination; and**
- **Medical decision making of low complexity.**

Counseling and/or coordination of care with other physicians, other qualified health care professionals, or agencies are provided consistent with the nature of the problem(s) and the patient's and/or family's needs.

Usually, the presenting problem(s) are of moderate severity. Typically, 30 minutes are spent face-to-face with the patient and/or family.

➲ *CPT Changes: An Insider's View* 2013

➲ *CPT Assistant* Winter 91:11, Spring 92:24, Summer 92:12, Spring 93:34, Spring 95:1, Jun 97:6, Nov 97:6-8, Oct 98:6, Jan 06:1, Jul 09:8, Aug 09:5, Jan 11:3, Jan 13:9, Jun 13:3

99343 **Home visit** for the evaluation and management of a new patient, which requires these 3 key components:

- **A detailed history;**
- **A detailed examination; and**
- **Medical decision making of moderate complexity.**

Counseling and/or coordination of care with other physicians, other qualified health care professionals, or agencies are provided consistent with the nature of the problem(s) and the patient's and/or family's needs.

Usually, the presenting problem(s) are of moderate to high severity. Typically, 45 minutes are spent face-to-face with the patient and/or family.

➲ *CPT Changes: An Insider's View* 2013

➲ *CPT Assistant* Winter 91:11, Spring 92:24, Summer 92:12, Spring 93:34, Spring 95:1, Jun 97:6, Nov 97:6-8, Oct 98:6, Jan 06:1, Jul 09:8, Aug 09:5, Jan 11:3, Jan 13:9, Jun 13:3

99344 **Home visit** for the evaluation and management of a new patient, which requires these 3 key components:

- **A comprehensive history;**
- **A comprehensive examination; and**
- **Medical decision making of moderate complexity.**

Counseling and/or coordination of care with other physicians, other qualified health care professionals, or agencies are provided consistent with the nature of the problem(s) and the patient's and/or family's needs.

Usually, the presenting problem(s) are of high severity. Typically, 60 minutes are spent face-to-face with the patient and/or family.

➲ *CPT Changes: An Insider's View* 2013

➲ *CPT Assistant* Nov 97:6-8, Oct 98:6, Jan 06:1, Jul 09:8, Aug 09:5, Jan 11:3, Jan 13:9, Jun 13:3

99345 **Home visit** for the evaluation and management of a new patient, which requires these 3 key components:

- **A comprehensive history;**
- **A comprehensive examination; and**
- **Medical decision making of high complexity.**

Counseling and/or coordination of care with other physicians, other qualified health care professionals, or agencies are provided consistent with the nature of the problem(s) and the patient's and/or family's needs.

Usually, the patient is unstable or has developed a significant new problem requiring immediate physician attention. Typically, 75 minutes are spent face-to-face with the patient and/or family.

➲ *CPT Changes: An Insider's View* 2013

➲ *CPT Assistant* Nov 97:6-8, Oct 98:6, Jan 06:1, Jul 09:8, Aug 09:5, Jan 11:3, Jan 12:3, Jan 13:9, Jun 13:3

Established Patient

99347 **Home visit** for the evaluation and management of an established patient, which requires at least 2 of these 3 key components:

- **A problem focused interval history;**
- **A problem focused examination;**
- **Straightforward medical decision making.**

Counseling and/or coordination of care with other physicians, other qualified health care professionals, or agencies are provided consistent with the nature of the problem(s) and the patient's and/or family's needs.

Usually, the presenting problem(s) are self limited or minor. Typically, 15 minutes are spent face-to-face with the patient and/or family.

➲ *CPT Changes: An Insider's View* 2013

➲ *CPT Assistant* Nov 97:6-8, Oct 98:6, May 05:1, Jan 06:1, Jul 07:1, Jul 09:8, Aug 09:5, Jan 11:3, Jan 12:3, Jan 13:9, Jun 13:3, Nov 13:3

99348 **Home visit** for the evaluation and management of an established patient, which requires at least 2 of these 3 key components:

- **An expanded problem focused interval history;**
- **An expanded problem focused examination;**
- **Medical decision making of low complexity.**

Counseling and/or coordination of care with other physicians, other qualified health care professionals, or agencies are provided consistent with the nature of the problem(s) and the patient's and/or family's needs.

Usually, the presenting problem(s) are of low to moderate severity. Typically, 25 minutes are spent face-to-face with the patient and/or family.

➲ *CPT Changes: An Insider's View* 2013

➲ *CPT Assistant* Nov 97:6-8, Oct 98:6, Jan 06:1, Jul 07:1, Jul 09:8, Aug 09:5, Jan 11:3, Jan 13:9, Jun 13:3

99349 **Home visit** for the evaluation and management of an established patient, which requires at least 2 of these 3 key components:

- **A detailed interval history;**
- **A detailed examination;**
- **Medical decision making of moderate complexity.**

Counseling and/or coordination of care with other physicians, other qualified health care professionals, or agencies are provided consistent with the nature of the problem(s) and the patient's and/or family's needs.

Usually, the presenting problem(s) are moderate to high severity. Typically, 40 minutes are spent face-to-face with the patient and/or family.

➲ *CPT Changes: An Insider's View* 2013

➲ *CPT Assistant* Nov 97:6-8, Oct 98:6, Jan 06:1, Jul 07:1, Jul 09:8, Aug 09:5, Jan 13:9, Jun 13:3

99350 **Home visit** for the evaluation and management of an established patient, which requires at least 2 of these 3 key components:

- **A comprehensive interval history;**
- **A comprehensive examination;**
- **Medical decision making of moderate to high complexity.**

Counseling and/or coordination of care with other physicians, other qualified health care professionals, or agencies are provided consistent with the nature of the problem(s) and the patient's and/or family's needs.

Usually, the presenting problem(s) are of moderate to high severity. The patient may be unstable or may have developed a significant new problem requiring immediate physician attention. Typically, 60 minutes are spent face-to-face with the patient and/or family.

➲ *CPT Changes: An Insider's View* 2013

➲ *CPT Assistant* Nov 97:6-8, Oct 98:6, Oct 03:7, Jan 06:1, Jul 07:1, Jul 09:8, Aug 09:5, Jan 12:3, Apr 12:10, Jan 13:9, Jun 13:3, Nov 13:3, Oct 14:3, Nov 14:14

Prolonged Services

▸Prolonged Service With Direct Patient Contact (Except with Office or Other Outpatient Services)◂

▸Codes 99354-99357 are used when a physician or other qualified health care professional provides prolonged service(s) involving direct patient contact that is provided beyond the usual service in either the inpatient, observation or outpatient setting, except with office or other outpatient services (99202, 99203, 99204, 99205, 99212, 99213, 99214, 99215). Direct patient contact is face-to-face and includes additional non-face-to-face services on the patient's floor or unit in the hospital or nursing facility during the same session. This service is reported in addition to the primary procedure. Appropriate codes should be selected for supplies provided or other procedures performed in the care of the patient during this period.

Codes 99354-99355 are used to report the total duration of face-to-face time spent by a physician or other qualified health care professional on a given date providing prolonged service in the outpatient setting, even if the time spent by the physician or other qualified health care professional on that date is not continuous. Codes 99356-99357 are used to report the total duration of time spent by a physician or other qualified health care professional at the bedside and on the patient's floor or unit in the hospital or nursing facility on a given date providing prolonged service to a patient, even if the time spent by the physician or other qualified health care professional on that date is not continuous.◀

Time spent performing separately reported services other than the E/M or psychotherapy service is not counted toward the prolonged services time.

Code 99354 or 99356 is used to report the first hour of prolonged service on a given date, depending on the place of service.

▶Either code should be used only once per date, even if the time spent by the physician or other qualified health care professional is not continuous on that date. Prolonged service of less than 30 minutes total duration on a given date is not separately reported.◀

Code 99355 or 99357 is used to report each additional 30 minutes beyond the first hour, depending on the place of service. Either code may also be used to report the final 15-30 minutes of prolonged service on a given date. Prolonged service of less than 15 minutes beyond the first hour or less than 15 minutes beyond the final 30 minutes is not reported separately.

The use of the time based add-on codes requires that the primary evaluation and management service have a typical or specified time published in the CPT codebook.

▶For E/M services that require prolonged clinical staff time and may include face-to-face services by the physician or other qualified health care professional, use 99415, 99416. Do not report 99354, 99355 with 99415, 99416, 99417.

For prolonged total time in addition to office or other outpatient services (ie, 99205, 99215), use 99417.

The following table illustrates the correct reporting of prolonged physician or other qualified health care professional service with direct patient contact in the inpatient or observation setting beyond the usual service time.◀

▶**Total Duration of Prolonged Services**	**Code(s)**
less than 30 minutes	Not reported separately
30-74 minutes (30 minutes - 1 hr. 14 min.)	99356 X 1
75-104 minutes (1 hr. 15 min. - 1 hr. 44 min.)	99356 X 1 AND 99357 X 1
105 minutes or more (1 hr. 45 min. or more)	99356 X 1 AND 99357 X 2 or more for each additional 30 minutes.◀

★+▲ **99354** Prolonged service(s) in the outpatient setting requiring direct patient contact beyond the time of the usual service; first hour (List separately in addition to code for outpatient **Evaluation and Management** or psychotherapy service, except with office or other outpatient services [99202, 99203, 99204, 99205, 99212, 99213, 99214, 99215])

➲ *CPT Changes: An Insider's View* 2009, 2012, 2016, 2017, 2021

➲ *CPT Assistant* Spring 94:30, 32, May 97:3, Sep 98:5, Sep 00:2, Jul 01:2, May 05:1, Nov 05:10, Jun 08:12, Sep 08:3, Jul 09:8, Apr 12:10, Aug 12:3, 4, 5, May 13:12, Jun 13:3, Oct 13:11, Apr 14:6, Jun 14:14, Oct 15:3, 9, Jun 19:7, Oct 19:10

►(Use 99354 in conjunction with 90837, 90847, 99241-99245, 99324-99337, 99341-99350, 99483)◄

►(Do not report 99354 in conjunction with 99202, 99203, 99204, 99205, 99212, 99213, 99214, 99215, 99415, 99416, 99417)◄

★+▲ **99355** each additional 30 minutes (List separately in addition to code for prolonged service)

➲ *CPT Changes: An Insider's View* 2009, 2012, 2016, 2017, 2021

➲ *CPT Assistant* Spring 94:30, 32, May 97:3, Sep 98:5, Sep 00:2, Jul 01:2, Nov 05:10, Jun 08:12, Sep 08:3, Jul 09:8, Apr 12:10, Aug 12:3, 4, 5, May 13:12, Jun 13:3, Oct 13:11, Apr 14:6, Jun 14:14, Oct 15:3, 9, Jun 19:7, Oct 19:10

(Use 99355 in conjunction with 99354)

►(Do not report 99355 in conjunction with 99202, 99203, 99204, 99205, 99212, 99213, 99214, 99215, 99415, 99416, 99417)◄

+▲ **99356** Prolonged service in the inpatient or observation setting, requiring unit/floor time beyond the usual service; first hour (List separately in addition to code for inpatient or observation **Evaluation and Management** service)

➲ *CPT Changes: An Insider's View* 2009, 2012, 2021

➲ *CPT Assistant* Spring 94:30, 32, Apr 97:3, May 97:3, Sep 98:5, Sep 00:2, Jul 01:2, Nov 05:10, Jun 08:12, Sep 08:3, Jul 09:8, Jun 11:3, Aug 11:11, Jul 12:11, Aug 12:3, 4, 5, May 13:12, Jun 13:3, Oct 13:11, Apr 14:6, Jun 14:14, Oct 15:3, 9, Jun 19:7

(Use 99356 in conjunction with 90837, 90847, 99218-99220, 99221-99223, 99224-99226, 99231-99233, 99234-99236, 99251-99255, 99304-99310)

+ **99357** each additional 30 minutes (List separately in addition to code for prolonged service)

➲ *CPT Changes: An Insider's View* 2009, 2012

➲ *CPT Assistant* Spring 94:34, Apr 97:3, May 97:3, Sep 98:5, Sep 00:2, Jul 01:2, Nov 05:10, Jun 08:12, Sep 08:3, Jul 09:8, Jun 11:3, Aug 11:11, Jul 12:11, Aug 12:3, 4, 5, May 13:12, Jun 13:3, Oct 13:11, Apr 14:6, Jun 14:14, Oct 15:3, 9, Jun 19:7

(Use 99357 in conjunction with 99356)

Prolonged Service Without Direct Patient Contact

►Codes 99358 and 99359 are used when a prolonged service is provided that is neither face-to-face time in the outpatient, inpatient, or observation setting, nor additional unit/floor time in the hospital or nursing facility setting. Codes 99358, 99359 may be used during the same session of an evaluation and management service, except office or other outpatient services (99202, 99203, 99204, 99205, 99212, 99213, 99214, 99215). For prolonged total time in addition to office or other outpatient services (ie, 99205, 99215) on the same date of service without direct patient contact, use 99417. Codes 99358, 99359 may also be used for prolonged services on a date other than the date of a face-to face encounter.

This service is to be reported in relation to other physician or other qualified health care professional services, including evaluation and management services at any level. This prolonged service may be reported on a different date than the primary service to which it is related. For example, extensive record review may relate to a previous evaluation and management service performed at an earlier date. However, it must relate to a service or patient where (face-to-face) patient care has occurred or will occur and relate to ongoing patient management.◄

Codes 99358 and 99359 are used to report the total duration of non-face-to-face time spent by a physician or other qualified health care professional on a given date providing prolonged service, even if the time spent by the physician or other qualified health care professional on that date is not continuous. Code 99358 is used to report the first hour of prolonged service on a given date regardless of the place of service. It should be used only once per date.

▶Prolonged service of less than 30 minutes total duration on a given date is not separately reported.

Code 99359 is used to report each additional 30 minutes beyond the first hour. It may also be used to report the final 15 to 30 minutes of prolonged service on a given date.◀

Prolonged service of less than 15 minutes beyond the first hour or less than 15 minutes beyond the final 30 minutes is not reported separately.

▶Do not report 99358, 99359 for time without direct patient contact reported in other services such as care plan oversight services (99339, 99340, 99374-99380), chronic care management by a physician or other qualified health care professional (99491), home and outpatient INR monitoring (93792, 93793), medical team conferences (99366-99368), interprofessional telephone/Internet/electronic health record consultations (99446, 99447, 99448, 99449, 99451, 99452), or online digital evaluation and management services (99421, 99422, 99423).◀

99358 **Prolonged evaluation and management service** before and/or after direct patient care; first hour

➲ *CPT Changes: An Insider's View* 2010, 2012

➲ *CPT Assistant* Spring 94:34, Nov 98:3, Sep 00:3, Nov 05:10, Jun 08:12, Sep 08:3, Aug 12:3, 4, 5, Apr 13:3, Oct 13:11, Nov 13:3, Oct 14:3, Oct 18:9, Jan 19:13, Jun 19:7

+ 99359 each additional 30 minutes (List separately in addition to code for prolonged service)

➲ *CPT Changes: An Insider's View* 2010, 2012

➲ *CPT Assistant* Spring 94:34, Sep 00:3, Nov 05:10, Jun 08:12, Sep 08:3, Aug 12:3, 4, 5, Apr 13:3, Oct 13:11, Nov 13:3, Oct 14:3, Oct 18:9, Jan 19:13, Jun 19:7

(Use 99359 in conjunction with 99358)

▶(Do not report 99358, 99359 on the same date of service as 99202, 99203, 99204, 99205, 99212, 99213, 99214, 99215, 99417)◀

Total Duration of Prolonged Services Without Direct Face-to-Face Contact	Code(s)
less than 30 minutes	Not reported separately
30-74 minutes (30 minutes - 1 hr. 14 min.)	99358 X 1
75-104 minutes (1 hr. 15 min. - 1 hr. 44 min.)	99358 X 1 AND 99359 X 1
105 minutes or more (1 hr. 45 min. or more)	99358 X 1 AND 99359 X 2 or more for each additional 30 minutes.

Prolonged Clinical Staff Services With Physician or Other Qualified Health Care Professional Supervision

►Codes 99415, 99416 are used when a prolonged evaluation and management (E/M) service is provided in the office or outpatient setting that involves prolonged clinical staff face-to-face time beyond the highest total time of the E/M service, as stated in the ranges of time in the code descriptions. The physician or qualified health care professional is present to provide direct supervision of the clinical staff. This service is reported in addition to the designated E/M services and any other services provided at the same session as E/M services.◄

Codes 99415, 99416 are used to report the total duration of face-to-face time spent by clinical staff on a given date providing prolonged service in the office or other outpatient setting, even if the time spent by the clinical staff on that date is not continuous. Time spent performing separately reported services other than the E/M service is not counted toward the prolonged services time.

►Code 99415 is used to report the first hour of prolonged clinical staff service on a given date. Code 99415 should be used only once per date, even if the time spent by the clinical staff is not continuous on that date. Prolonged service of less than 30 minutes total duration on a given date is not separately reported because the clinical staff time involved is included in the E/M codes. The highest total time in the time ranges of the code descriptions is used in defining when prolonged services time begins. For example, prolonged clinical staff services for 99214 begin after 39 minutes, and 99415 is not reported until at least 69 minutes total face-to-face clinical staff time has been performed. When face-to-face time is noncontiguous, use only the face-to-face time provided to the patient by the clinical staff.◄

Code 99416 is used to report each additional 30 minutes of prolonged clinical staff service beyond the first hour. Code 99416 may also be used to report the final 15-30 minutes of prolonged service on a given date. Prolonged service of less than 15 minutes beyond the first hour or less than 15 minutes beyond the final 30 minutes is not reported separately.

►Codes 99415, 99416 may be reported for no more than two simultaneous patients. The use of the time-based add-on codes requires that the primary E/M service has a time published in the CPT code set.

For prolonged services by the physician or other qualified health care professional, see 99354, 99355, 99417. Do not report 99415, 99416 with 99354, 99355, 99417.◄

Facilities may not report 99415, 99416.

#+▲ 99415 Prolonged clinical staff service (the service beyond the highest time in the range of total time of the service) during an evaluation and management service in the office or outpatient setting, direct patient contact with physician supervision; first hour (List separately in addition to code for outpatient **Evaluation and Management** service)

➲ *CPT Changes: An Insider's View* 2016, 2021

➲ *CPT Assistant* Oct 15:3, Feb 16:13, Oct 19:10

►(Use 99415 in conjunction with 99202, 99203, 99204, 99205, 99212, 99213, 99214, 99215)◄

►(Do not report 99415 in conjunction with 99354, 99355, 99417)◄

#+▲ 99416 each additional 30 minutes (List separately in addition to code for prolonged service)

➲ *CPT Changes: An Insider's View* 2016, 2021

➲ *CPT Assistant* Oct 15:3, Feb 16:13, Oct 19:10

(Use 99416 in conjunction with 99415)

►(Do not report 99416 in conjunction with 99354, 99355, 99417)◄

E/M 99202-99499

▶The Total Duration of Prolonged Services Table illustrates the correct reporting of prolonged services provided by clinical staff with physician supervision in the office setting beyond the initial 30 minutes of clinical staff time:

Total Duration of Prolonged Services	Code(s)
less than 30 minutes	Not reported separately
30-74 minutes (30 minutes - 1 hr. 14 min.)	99415 X 1
75-104 minutes (1 hr. 15 min. - 1 hr. 44 min.)	99415 X 1 AND 99416 X 1
105 minutes or more (1 hr. 45 min. or more)	99415 X 1 AND 99416 X 2 or more for each additional 30 minutes.◀

▶Prolonged Service With or Without Direct Patient Contact on the Date of an Office or Other Outpatient Service◀

▶Code 99417 is used to report prolonged total time (ie, combined time with and without direct patient contact) provided by the physician or other qualified health care professional on the date of office or other outpatient services (ie, 99205, 99215). Code 99417 is only used when the office or other outpatient service has been selected using time alone as the basis and only after the minimum time required to report the highest-level service (ie, 99205 or 99215) has been exceeded by 15 minutes. To report a unit of 99417, 15 minutes of additional time must have been attained. Do not report 99417 for any additional time increment of less than 15 minutes.

The listed time ranges for 99205 (ie, 60-74 minutes) and 99215 (ie, 40-54 minutes) represent the complete range of time for which each code may be reported. Therefore, when reporting 99417, the initial time unit of 15 minutes should be added once the minimum time in the primary E/M code has been surpassed by 15 minutes. For example, to report the initial unit of 99417 for a new patient encounter (99205), do not report 99417 until at least 15 minutes of time has been accumulated beyond 60 minutes (ie, 75 minutes) on the date of the encounter. For an established patient encounter (99215), do not report 99417 until at least 15 minutes of time has been accumulated beyond 40 minutes (ie, 55 minutes) on the date of the encounter.

Time spent performing separately reported services other than the E/M service is not counted toward the time to report 99205, 99215 and prolonged services time.

For prolonged services on a date other than the date of a face-to-face encounter, including office or other outpatient services (99202, 99203, 99204, 99205, 99212, 99213, 99214, 99215), see 99358, 99359. For E/M services that require prolonged clinical staff time and may include face-to-face services by the physician or other QHP, see 99415, 99416. Do not report 99417 in conjunction with 99354, 99355, 99358, 99359, 99415, 99416.

Prolonged services of less than 15 minutes total time is not reported on the date of office or other outpatient service when the highest level is reached (ie, 99205, 99215).◀

#★+● **99417** Prolonged office or other outpatient evaluation and management service(s) beyond the minimum required time of the primary procedure which has been selected using total time, requiring total time with or without direct patient contact beyond the usual service, on the date of the primary service, each 15 minutes of total time (List separately in addition to codes 99205, 99215 for office or other outpatient **Evaluation and Management** services)

➲ *CPT Changes: An Insider's View* 2021

▶(Use 99417 in conjunction with 99205, 99215)◀

▶(Do not report 99417 on the same date of service as 99354, 99355, 99358, 99359, 99415, 99416)◀

▶(Do not report 99417 for any time unit less than 15 minutes)◀

▶**Total Duration of New Patient Office or Other Outpatient Services (use with 99205)**	**Code(s)**
less than 75 minutes	Not reported separately
75-89 minutes	99205 X 1 and 99417 X 1
90-104 minutes	99205 X 1 and 99417 X 2
105 minutes or more	99205 X 1 and 99417 X 3 or more for each additional 15 minutes

Total Duration of Established Patient Office or Other Outpatient Services (use with 99215)	**Code(s)**
less than 55 minutes	Not reported separately
55-69 minutes	99215 X 1 and 99417 X 1
70-84 minutes	99215 X 1 and 99417 X 2
85 minutes or more	99215 X 1 and 99417 X 3 or more for each additional 15 minutes◀

Standby Services

Code 99360 is used to report physician or other qualified health care professional standby services that are requested by another individual and that involve prolonged attendance without direct (face-to-face) patient contact. Care or services may not be provided to other patients during this period. This code is not used to report time spent proctoring another individual. It is also not used if the period of standby ends with the performance of a procedure, subject to a surgical package by the individual who was on standby.

Code 99360 is used to report the total duration of time spent on a given date on standby. Standby service of less than 30 minutes total duration on a given date is not reported separately.

Second and subsequent periods of standby beyond the first 30 minutes may be reported only if a full 30 minutes of standby was provided for each unit of service reported.

99360 **Standby service,** requiring prolonged attendance, each 30 minutes (eg, operative standby, standby for frozen section, for cesarean/high risk delivery, for monitoring EEG)

➲ *CPT Changes: An Insider's View* 2013

➲ *CPT Assistant* Spring 94:32, Apr 97:10, Aug 97:18, Nov 97:8, Nov 99:5-6, Aug 00:3, Sep 00:3, May 05:1, Nov 05:10, Nov 06:23, Mar 08:14, Feb 11:3, May 13:8, Apr 14:5, 11

(For hospital mandated on call services, see 99026, 99027)

(99360 may be reported in addition to 99460, 99465 as appropriate)

(Do not report 99360 in conjunction with 99464)

Case Management Services

Case management is a process in which a physician or another qualified health care professional is responsible for direct care of a patient and, additionally, for coordinating, managing access to, initiating, and/or supervising other health care services needed by the patient.

Anticoagulant Management

(99363, 99364 have been deleted. To report, see 93792, 93793)

Medical Team Conferences

Medical team conferences include face-to-face participation by a minimum of three qualified health care professionals from different specialties or disciplines (each of whom provide direct care to the patient), with or without the presence of the patient, family member(s), community agencies, surrogate decision maker(s) (eg, legal guardian), and/or caregiver(s). The participants are actively involved in the development, revision, coordination, and implementation of health care services needed by the patient. Reporting participants shall have performed face-to-face evaluations or treatments of the patient, independent of any team conference, within the previous 60 days.

Physicians or other qualified health care professionals who may report evaluation and management services should report their time spent in a team conference with the patient and/or family present using evaluation and management (E/M) codes (and time as the key controlling factor for code selection when counseling and/or coordination of care dominates the service). These introductory guidelines do not apply to services reported using E/M codes (see E/M services guidelines). However, the individual must be directly involved with the patient, providing face-to-face services outside of the conference visit with other physicians, and qualified health care professionals, or agencies.

Reporting participants shall document their participation in the team conference as well as their contributed information and subsequent treatment recommendations.

No more than one individual from the same specialty may report 99366-99368 at the same encounter.

Individuals should not report 99366-99368 when their participation in the medical team conference is part of a facility or organizational service contractually provided by the organization or facility.

The team conference starts at the beginning of the review of an individual patient and ends at the conclusion of the review. Time related to record keeping and report generation is not reported. The reporting participant shall be present for all time reported. The time reported is not limited to the time that the participant is communicating to the other team members or patient and/or family. Time reported for medical team conferences may not be used in the determination of time for other services such as care plan oversight (99374-99380), home, domiciliary, or rest home care plan oversight (99339-99340), prolonged services (99354-99359), psychotherapy, or any E/M service. For team conferences where the patient is present for any part of the duration of the conference, nonphysician qualified health care professionals (eg, speech-language pathologists, physical therapists, occupational therapists, social workers, dietitians) report the team conference face-to-face code 99366.

►Comparison of Prolonged Services Codes (99354, 99355, 99356, 99357, 99358, 99359, 99417) Table◄

►Code	Patient Contact	Minimum Reportable Prolonged Services Time (Single Date of Service)	Use In Conjunction With	*Do Not Report With	Other Prolonged Service(s) Reportable On Same Date Of Service
+99354	Face-to-Face Only	30 minutes (Beyond listed typical time)	90837, 90847, 99241-99245, 99324-99337, 99341-99350, 99483	99202-99205, 99212-99215, 99415, 99416, 99417	99358, 99359
+99355	Face-to-Face Only	Each additional 15 minutes (Beyond 99354)	99354	99202-99205, 99212-99215, 99415, 99416, 99417	99358, 99359
+99356	Face-to-Face and Unit/Floor Time	30 minutes (Beyond listed typical time)	90837, 90847, 99218-99220, 99221-99223, 99224-99226, 99231-99233, 99234-99236, 99251-99255, 99304-99310		99358, 99359
+99357	Face-to-Face and Unit/Floor Time	Each additional 15 minutes (Beyond 99356)	99356		99358, 99359
99358	Non-Face-to-Face Only	30 minutes	Must relate to a service where face-to-face care has or will occur. This is not an add-on code and is not used in conjunction with a base code.	99202-99205, 99212-99215, 99417 On same date of service	99354, 99356
+99359	Non-Face-to-Face Only	Each additional 15 minutes (Beyond 99358)	99358	99202-99205, 99212-99215, 99417 On same date of service	99354, 99356
+99417	Face-to-Face and/or Non-Face-to-Face	Reported with 99205: 75 minutes or more Reported with 99215: 55 minutes or more ***(Total time on the date of encounter)***	99205, 99215	99354, 99355, 99358, 99359, 99415, 99416	N/A

*Do not count the time of any separately reported service as prolonged services time
99355 is for prolonged services time beyond 99354 and may be reported in multiple units
99357 is for prolonged services time beyond 99356 and may be reported in multiple units
99359 is for prolonged services time beyond 99358 and may be reported in multiple units
99417 is for prolonged services time beyond 99205 or 99215 and may be reported in multiple units of at least 15 minutes◄

Medical Team Conference, Direct (Face-to-Face) Contact With Patient and/or Family

99366 **Medical team conference** with interdisciplinary team of health care professionals, face-to-face with patient and/or family, 30 minutes or more, participation by nonphysician qualified health care professional

➲ *CPT Changes: An Insider's View* 2008

➲ *CPT Assistant* Apr 13:3, Jun 14:3, Oct 14:3

(Team conference services of less than 30 minutes duration are not reported separately)

(For team conference services by a physician with patient and/or family present, see Evaluation and Management services)

►(Do not report 99366 during the same month with 99439, 99487, 99489, 99490, 99491)◄

Medical Team Conference, Without Direct (Face-to-Face) Contact With Patient and/or Family

99367 **Medical team conference** with interdisciplinary team of health care professionals, patient and/or family not present, 30 minutes or more; participation by physician

➲ *CPT Changes: An Insider's View* 2008

➲ *CPT Assistant* Apr 13:3, Jun 14:3, Dec 19:14

99368 participation by nonphysician qualified health care professional

➲ *CPT Changes: An Insider's View* 2008

➲ *CPT Assistant* Apr 13:3, Jun 14:3, Oct 14:3

(Team conference services of less than 30 minutes duration are not reported separately)

►(Do not report 99367, 99368 during the same month with 99439, 99487, 99489, 99490, 99491)◄

Care Plan Oversight Services

Care plan oversight services are reported separately from codes for office/outpatient, hospital, home, nursing facility or domiciliary, or non-face-to-face services. The complexity and approximate time of the care plan oversight services provided within a 30-day period determine code selection. Only one individual may report services for a given period of time, to reflect the sole or predominant supervisory role with a particular patient. These codes should not be reported for supervision of patients in nursing facilities or under the care of home health agencies unless they require recurrent supervision of therapy.

The work involved in providing very low intensity or infrequent supervision services is included in the pre- and post-encounter work for home, office/outpatient and nursing facility or domiciliary visit codes.

(For care plan oversight services of patients in the home, domiciliary, or rest home [eg, assisted living facility], see 99339, 99340, and for hospice agency, see 99377, 99378)

(Do not report 99374-99380 for time reported with 98966, 98967, 98968, 99421, 99422, 99423, 99441, 99442, 99443)

(Do not report 99374-99378 during the same month with 99487-99489)

99374 **Supervision** of a patient under care of home health agency (patient not present) in home, domiciliary or equivalent environment (eg, Alzheimer's facility) requiring complex and multidisciplinary care modalities involving regular development and/or revision of care plans by that individual, review of subsequent reports of patient status, review of related laboratory and other studies, communication (including telephone calls) for purposes of assessment or care decisions with health care professional(s), family member(s), surrogate decision maker(s) (eg, legal guardian) and/or key caregiver(s) involved in patient's care, integration of new information into the medical treatment plan and/or adjustment of medical therapy, within a calendar month; 15-29 minutes

➲ *CPT Changes: An Insider's View* 2002, 2013

➲ *CPT Assistant* Summer 94:9, Nov 97:8-9, May 05:1, Dec 06:4, Mar 07:11, Mar 08:6, Sep 08:3, Jul 09:5, 10, Apr 13:3, Jul 13:11, Sep 13:15, Nov 13:3, Feb 14:11, Oct 14:3

99375 30 minutes or more

➲ *CPT Changes: An Insider's View* 2013

➲ *CPT Assistant* Summer 94:9, Nov 97:8-9, Dec 06:4, Mar 07:11, Mar 08:6, Sep 08:3, Jul 09:5, 10, Apr 13:3, Jul 13:11, Sep 13:15

99377 **Supervision** of a hospice patient (patient not present) requiring complex and multidisciplinary care modalities involving regular development and/or revision of care plans by that individual, review of subsequent reports of patient status, review of related laboratory and other studies, communication (including telephone calls) for purposes of assessment or care decisions with health care professional(s), family member(s), surrogate decision maker(s) (eg, legal guardian) and/or key caregiver(s) involved in patient's care, integration of new information into the medical treatment plan and/or adjustment of medical therapy, within a calendar month; 15-29 minutes

➲ *CPT Changes: An Insider's View* 2001, 2002, 2013

➲ *CPT Assistant* Nov 97:8-9, Dec 06:4, Mar 07:11, Sep 08:3, Jul 09:5, 10, Apr 13:3, Jul 13:11, Sep 13:15

99378 30 minutes or more

➲ *CPT Changes: An Insider's View* 2013

➲ *CPT Assistant* Nov 97:8-9, Dec 06:4, Mar 07:11, Mar 08:6, Sep 08:3, Jul 09:5, 10, Apr 13:3, Jul 13:11, Sep 13:15

99379 **Supervision** of a nursing facility patient (patient not present) requiring complex and multidisciplinary care modalities involving regular development and/or revision of care plans by that individual, review of subsequent reports of patient status, review of related laboratory and other studies, communication (including telephone calls) for purposes of assessment or care decisions with health care professional(s), family member(s), surrogate decision maker(s) (eg, legal guardian) and/or key caregiver(s) involved in patient's care, integration of new information into the medical treatment plan and/or adjustment of medical therapy, within a calendar month; 15-29 minutes

➲ *CPT Changes: An Insider's View* 2002, 2013

➲ *CPT Assistant* Dec 06:4, Mar 08:6, Sep 08:3, Jul 09:5, Apr 13:3, Jul 13:11, Sep 13:15

99380 30 minutes or more

➲ *CPT Changes: An Insider's View* 2013

➲ *CPT Assistant* Nov 97:8-9, Dec 06:4, Mar 08:6, Sep 08:3, Jul 09:5, Apr 13:3, Jul 13:11, Sep 13:15, Nov 13:3, Oct 14:3

Preventive Medicine Services

The following codes are used to report the preventive medicine evaluation and management of infants, children, adolescents, and adults.

The extent and focus of the services will largely depend on the age of the patient.

►If an abnormality is encountered or a preexisting problem is addressed in the process of performing this preventive medicine evaluation and management service, and if the problem or abnormality is significant enough to require additional work to perform the key components of a problem-oriented evaluation and management service, then the appropriate office/outpatient code 99202, 99203, 99204, 99205, 99211, 99212, 99213, 99214, 99215 should also be reported. Modifier 25 should be added to the office/outpatient code to indicate that a significant, separately identifiable evaluation and management service was provided on the same day as the preventive medicine service. The appropriate preventive medicine service is additionally reported.◀

An insignificant or trivial problem/abnormality that is encountered in the process of performing the preventive medicine evaluation and management service and which does not require additional work and the performance of the key components of a problem-oriented E/M service should not be reported.

▶The "comprehensive" nature of the preventive medicine services codes 99381-99397 reflects an age- and gender- appropriate history/exam and is **not** synonymous with the "comprehensive" examination required in evaluation and management codes 99202-99350.◀

Codes 99381-99397 include counseling/anticipatory guidance/risk factor reduction interventions which are provided at the time of the initial or periodic comprehensive preventive medicine examination. (Refer to 99401, 99402, 99403, 99404, 99411, and 99412 for reporting those counseling/anticipatory guidance/risk factor reduction interventions that are provided at an encounter separate from the preventive medicine examination.)

(For behavior change intervention, see 99406, 99407, 99408, 99409)

Vaccine/toxoid products, immunization administrations, ancillary studies involving laboratory, radiology, other procedures, or screening tests (eg, vision, hearing, developmental) identified with a specific CPT code are reported separately. For immunization administration and vaccine risk/benefit counseling, see 90460, 90461, 90471-90474. For vaccine/toxoid products, see 90476-90749.

New Patient

99381 **Initial comprehensive preventive medicine** evaluation and management of an individual including an age and gender appropriate history, examination, counseling/anticipatory guidance/risk factor reduction interventions, and the ordering of laboratory/diagnostic procedures, new patient; infant (age younger than 1 year)

➲ *CPT Changes: An Insider's View* 2002, 2009

➲ *CPT Assistant* Winter 91:11, Spring 93:14, 34, Spring 95:1, Aug 97:1, Jul 98:9, Sep 98:5, Nov 98:3-4, May 02:1, May 05:1, Aug 05:15, Oct 06:15, Mar 09:3, Jul 09:7, Aug 09:5, Jan 13:9, Dec 14:18, Mar 16:7

99382 early childhood (age 1 through 4 years)

➲ *CPT Changes: An Insider's View* 2009

➲ *CPT Assistant* Winter 91:11, Spring 93:14, 34, Spring 95:1, Aug 97:1, Jul 98:9, Sep 98:5, Nov 98:3-4, May 02:1, Aug 05:15, Oct 06:15, Jul 09:5, Aug 09:5, Jan 13:9, Dec 14:18, Mar 16:7

99383 late childhood (age 5 through 11 years)

➲ *CPT Changes: An Insider's View* 2009

➲ *CPT Assistant* Winter 91:11, Spring 93:14, 34, Spring 95:1, Aug 97:1, Jul 98:9, Sep 98:5, Nov 98:3-4, May 02:1, Aug 05:15, Oct 06:15, Jul 09:7, Aug 09:5, Jan 13:9, Dec 14:18, Mar 16:7

99384 adolescent (age 12 through 17 years)

➲ *CPT Changes: An Insider's View* 2009

➲ *CPT Assistant* Winter 91:11, Spring 93:14, 34, Spring 95:1, Aug 97:1, Jul 98:9, Sep 98:5, Nov 98:3-4, May 02:1, Aug 05:15, Oct 06:15, Jul 09:7, Aug 09:5, Jan 13:9, Dec 14:18, Jan 15:12, Mar 16:7

99385 18-39 years

➲ *CPT Changes: An Insider's View* 2009

➲ *CPT Assistant* Winter 91:11, Spring 93:14, 34, Spring 95:1, Aug 97:7, Jul 98:9, Sep 98:5, Nov 98:3-4, May 02:1, Aug 05:15, Oct 06:15, Jul 09:5, Aug 09:5, Jan 13:9, Dec 14:18, Jan 15:12, Mar 16:7

99386 40-64 years

➲ *CPT Changes: An Insider's View* 2009

➲ *CPT Assistant* Winter 91:11, Spring 93:14, 34, Spring 95:1, Aug 97:1, Jul 98:9, Sep 98:5, Nov 98:3-4, May 02:1, Aug 05:15, Oct 06:15, Jul 09:7, Aug 09:5, Jan 13:9, Dec 14:18, Jan 15:12, Mar 16:7

99387 65 years and older

➲ *CPT Changes: An Insider's View* 2009

➲ *CPT Assistant* Winter 91:11, Spring 93:14, 34, Spring 95:1, Aug 97:1, Jul 98:9, Sep 98:5, Nov 98:3-4, May 02:1, Aug 05:15, Oct 06:15, Jul 09:7, Aug 09:5, Jan 13:9, Dec 14:18, Mar 16:7

Established Patient

99391 **Periodic comprehensive preventive medicine** reevaluation and management of an individual including an age and gender appropriate history, examination, counseling/anticipatory guidance/risk factor reduction interventions, and the ordering of laboratory/diagnostic procedures, established patient; infant (age younger than 1 year)

➲ *CPT Changes: An Insider's View* 2002, 2009

➲ *CPT Assistant* Winter 91:11, Spring 93:14, 34, Spring 95:1, Aug 97:1, Jul 98:9, Sep 98:5, Nov 98:3-4, May 02:1, May 05:1, Aug 05:15, Oct 06:15, Mar 09:3, Jul 09:7, Aug 09:5, Jan 13:9, Dec 14:18, Mar 16:7

99392 early childhood (age 1 through 4 years)

➲ *CPT Changes: An Insider's View* 2009

➲ *CPT Assistant* Winter 91:11, Spring 93:14, 34, Spring 95:1, Aug 97:1, Jul 98:9, Sep 98:5, Nov 98:3-4, May 02:1, Aug 05:15, Oct 06:15, Jul 09:7, Jan 13:9, Dec 14:18, Mar 16:7

99393 late childhood (age 5 through 11 years)

➲ *CPT Changes: An Insider's View* 2009

➲ *CPT Assistant* Winter 91:11, Spring 93:14, 34, Spring 95:1, Aug 97:1, Jul 98:9, Sep 98:5, Nov 98:3-4, May 02:1, Aug 05:15, Oct 06:15, Jul 09:7, Jan 13:9, Dec 14:18, Mar 16:7

99394 adolescent (age 12 through 17 years)

➲ *CPT Changes: An Insider's View* 2009

➲ *CPT Assistant* Winter 91:11, Spring 93:14, 34, Spring 95:1, Aug 97:1, Jul 98:9, Sep 98:5, Nov 98:3-4, May 02:1, Aug 05:15, Oct 06:15, Jul 09:7, Jan 13:9, Dec 14:18, Jan 15:12, Mar 16:7

99395 18-39 years

➲ *CPT Changes: An Insider's View* 2009

➲ *CPT Assistant* Winter 91:11, Spring 93:14, 34, Spring 95:1, Aug 97:1, Jul 98:9, Sep 98:5, Nov 98:3-4, May 02:1, Aug 05:15, Oct 06:15, Mar 08:3, Jul 09:7, Jan 13:9, Dec 14:18, Jan 15:12, Mar 16:7

99396 40-64 years

➲ *CPT Changes: An Insider's View* 2009

➲ *CPT Assistant* Winter 91:11, Spring 93:14, 34, Spring 95:1, Aug 97:1, Jul 98:9, Sep 98:5, Nov 98:3-4, May 02:1, Aug 05:15, Oct 06:15, Jul 09:7, Mar 12:4, Jan 13:9, Dec 14:18, Jan 15:12, Mar 16:7, Sep 17:11

99397 65 years and older

➲ *CPT Changes: An Insider's View* 2009

➲ *CPT Assistant* Winter 91:11, Spring 93:14, 34, Spring 95:1, Aug 97:1, Jul 98:9, Sep 98:5, Nov 98:3-4, May 02:1, Aug 05:15, Oct 06:15, Jul 09:7, Jan 13:9, Dec 14:18, Mar 16:7

Counseling Risk Factor Reduction and Behavior Change Intervention

New or Established Patient

These codes are used to report services provided face-to-face by a physician or other qualified health care professional for the purpose of promoting health and preventing illness or injury. They are distinct from evaluation and management (E/M) services that may be reported separately with modifier 25 when performed. Risk factor reduction services are used for persons without a specific illness for which the counseling might otherwise be used as part of treatment.

Preventive medicine counseling and risk factor reduction interventions will vary with age and should address such issues as family problems, diet and exercise, substance use, sexual practices, injury prevention, dental health, and diagnostic and laboratory test results available at the time of the encounter.

Behavior change interventions are for persons who have a behavior that is often considered an illness itself, such as tobacco use and addiction, substance abuse/misuse, or obesity. Behavior change services may be reported when performed as part of the treatment of condition(s) related to or potentially exacerbated by the behavior or when performed to change the harmful behavior that has not yet resulted in illness. Any E/M services reported on the same day must be distinct and reported with modifier 25, and time spent providing these services may not be used as a basis for the E/M code selection. Behavior change services involve specific validated interventions of assessing readiness for change and barriers to change, advising a change in behavior, assisting by providing specific suggested actions and motivational counseling, and arranging for services and follow-up.

For counseling groups of patients with symptoms or established illness, use 99078.

Health behavior assessment and intervention services (96156, 96158, 96159, 96164, 96165, 96167, 96168, 96170, 96171) should not be reported on the same day as codes 99401-99412.

Preventive Medicine, Individual Counseling

99401 **Preventive medicine counseling** and/or risk factor reduction intervention(s) provided to an individual (separate procedure); approximately 15 minutes

➲ *CPT Assistant* Aug 97:1, Jan 98:12, May 05:1, Aug 07:9, Oct 10:3, Dec 10:3, Jan 13:9, Aug 14:5, Mar 16:7

99402 approximately 30 minutes

➲ *CPT Assistant* Aug 97:1, Jan 98:12, May 05:1, Oct 10:3, Dec 10:3, Jan 13:9, Mar 16:7

99403 approximately 45 minutes

➲ *CPT Assistant* Aug 97:1, Jan 98:12, May 05:1, Oct 10:3, Dec 10:3, Jan 13:9, Mar 16:7

99404 approximately 60 minutes

➲ *CPT Assistant* Aug 97:1, Jan 98:12, May 05:1, Oct 10:3, Dec 10:3, Jan 13:9, Aug 14:5, Mar 16:7

Behavior Change Interventions, Individual

★ **99406** Smoking and tobacco use cessation counseling visit; intermediate, greater than 3 minutes up to 10 minutes

➲ *CPT Changes: An Insider's View* 2008, 2017

➲ *CPT Assistant* Jan 08:1, Sep 09:11, Oct 10:3, Dec 10:3, Jan 13:9, Mar 16:7

★ **99407** intensive, greater than 10 minutes

➲ *CPT Changes: An Insider's View* 2008, 2017

➲ *CPT Assistant* Jan 08:1, Sep 09:11, Oct 10:3, Dec 10:3, Jan 13:9, Mar 16:7

(Do not report 99407 in conjunction with 99406)

★ **99408** Alcohol and/or substance (other than tobacco) abuse structured screening (eg, AUDIT, DAST), and brief intervention (SBI) services; 15 to 30 minutes

➲ *CPT Changes: An Insider's View* 2008, 2017

➲ *CPT Assistant* Oct 10:3, Dec 10:3, Jan 13:9, Mar 16:7, Nov 16:5

(Do not report services of less than 15 minutes with 99408)

★ **99409** greater than 30 minutes
➔ *CPT Changes: An Insider's View* 2008, 2017
➔ *CPT Assistant* Oct 10:3, Dec 10:3, Jan 13:9, Mar 16:7, Nov 16:5

(Do not report 99409 in conjunction with 99408)

(Do not report 99408, 99409 in conjunction with 96160, 96161)

(Use 99408, 99409 only for initial screening and brief intervention)

Preventive Medicine, Group Counseling

99411 **Preventive medicine counseling** and/or risk factor reduction intervention(s) provided to individuals in a group setting (separate procedure); approximately 30 minutes
➔ *CPT Assistant* Aug 97:1, Jan 98:12, Sep 98:5, May 05:1, Oct 10:3, Dec 10:3, Jan 13:9, Mar 16:7

99412 approximately 60 minutes
➔ *CPT Assistant* Aug 97:1, Jan 98:12, Sep 98:5, May 05:1, Aug 07:9, Oct 10:3, Dec 10:3, Jan 13:9, Mar 16:7

99415 Code is out of numerical sequence. See 99358-99366

99416 Code is out of numerical sequence. See 99358-99366

99417 Code is out of numerical sequence. See 99358-99366

Other Preventive Medicine Services

99421 Code is out of numerical sequence. See 99442-99447

99422 Code is out of numerical sequence. See 99442-99447

99423 Code is out of numerical sequence. See 99442-99447

99429 **Unlisted preventive** medicine service
➔ *CPT Assistant* Sep 98:5, May 05:1, Oct 10:3, Dec 10:3, Jan 13:9, Mar 16:7

Non-Face-to-Face Services

Telephone Services

Telephone services are non-face-to-face evaluation and management (E/M) services provided to a patient using the telephone by a physician or other qualified health care professional, who may report evaluation and management services. These codes are used to report episodes of patient care initiated by an established patient or guardian of an established patient. If the telephone service ends with a decision to see the patient within 24 hours or next available urgent visit appointment, the code is not reported; rather the encounter is considered part of the preservice work of the subsequent E/M service, procedure, and visit. Likewise, if the telephone call refers to an E/M service performed and reported by that individual within the previous seven days (either requested or unsolicited patient follow-up) or within the postoperative period of the previously completed procedure, then the service(s) is considered part of that previous E/M service or procedure. (Do not report 99441-99443, if 99421, 99422, 99423 have been reported by the same provider in the previous seven days for the same problem.)

(For telephone services provided by a qualified nonphysician who may not report evaluation and management services [eg, speech-language pathologists, physical therapists, occupational therapists, social workers, dietitians], see 98966-98968)

99439 Code is out of numerical sequence. See 99480-99489

99441 Telephone evaluation and management service by a physician or other qualified health care professional who may report evaluation and management services provided to an established patient, parent, or guardian not originating from a related E/M service provided within the previous 7 days nor leading to an E/M service or procedure within the next 24 hours or soonest available appointment; 5-10 minutes of medical discussion

➲ *CPT Changes: An Insider's View* 2008, 2013

➲ *CPT Assistant* Mar 08:6, Apr 13:3, Oct 13:11, Nov 13:3, Oct 14:3, Mar 18:7, Jan 19:13, Mar 19:8

99442 11-20 minutes of medical discussion

➲ *CPT Changes: An Insider's View* 2008, 2013

➲ *CPT Assistant* Mar 08:6, Apr 13:3, Oct 13:11, Mar 18:7, Jan 19:13, Mar 19:8

99443 21-30 minutes of medical discussion

➲ *CPT Changes: An Insider's View* 2008, 2013

➲ *CPT Assistant* Mar 08:6, Apr 13:3, Oct 13:11, Nov 13:3, Oct 14:3, Mar 18:7, Jan 19:13, Mar 19:8

(Do not report 99441-99443 when using 99339-99340, 99374-99380 for the same call[s])

(Do not report 99441-99443 for home and outpatient INR monitoring when reporting 93792, 93793)

(Do not report 99441-99443 during the same month with 99487-99489)

(Do not report 99441-99443 when performed during the service time of codes 99495 or 99496)

Online Digital Evaluation and Management Services

Online digital evaluation and management (E/M) services (99421, 99422, 99423) are patient-initiated services with physicians or other qualified health care professionals (QHPs). Online digital E/M services require physician or other QHP's evaluation, assessment, and management of the patient. These services are not for the nonevaluative electronic communication of test results, scheduling of appointments, or other communication that does not include E/M. While the patient's problem may be new to the physician or other QHP, the patient is an established patient. Patients initiate these services through Health Insurance Portability and Accountability Act (HIPAA)-compliant secure platforms, such as electronic health record (EHR) portals, secure email, or other digital applications, which allow digital communication with the physician or other QHP.

Online digital E/M services are reported once for the physician's or other QHP's cumulative time devoted to the service during a seven-day period. The seven-day period begins with the physician's or other QHP's initial, personal review of the patient-generated inquiry. Physician's or other QHP's cumulative service time includes review of the initial inquiry, review of patient records or data pertinent to assessment of the patient's problem, personal physician or other QHP interaction with clinical staff focused on the patient's problem, development of management plans, including physician- or other QHP generation of prescriptions or ordering of tests, and subsequent communication with the patient through online, telephone, email, or other digitally supported communication, which does not otherwise represent a separately reported E/M service. All professional decision making, assessment, and subsequent management by physicians or other QHPs in the same group practice contribute to the cumulative service time of the patient's online digital E/M service. Online digital E/M services require permanent documentation storage (electronic or hard copy) of the encounter.

If within seven days of the initiation of an online digital E/M service, a separately reported E/M visit occurs, then the physician or other QHP work devoted to the online digital E/M service is incorporated into the separately reported E/M visit (eg, additive of visit time for a time-based E/M visit or additive of decision-making complexity for a key component-based E/M visit). This includes E/M visits and procedures that are provided through synchronous telemedicine visits using interactive audio and video telecommunication equipment, which are reported with modifier 95 appended to the

E/M service code. If the patient initiates an online digital inquiry for the same or a related problem within seven days of a previous E/M service, then the online digital visit is not reported. If the online digital inquiry is related to a surgical procedure and occurs during the postoperative period of a previously completed procedure, then the online digital E/M service is not reported separately. If the patient generates the initial online digital inquiry for a new problem within seven days of a previous E/M visit that addressed a different problem, then the online digital E/M service may be reported separately. If the patient presents a new, unrelated problem during the seven-day period of an online digital E/M service, then the physician's or other QHP's time spent on evaluation, assessment, and management of the additional problem is added to the cumulative service time of the online digital E/M service for that seven-day period.

(For online digital E/M services provided by a qualified nonphysician health care professional who may not report the physician or other qualified health care professional E/M services [eg, speech-language pathologists, physical therapists, occupational therapists, social workers, dietitians], see 98970, 98971, 98972)

 # 99421 Online digital evaluation and management service, for an established patient, for up to 7 days, cumulative time during the 7 days; 5-10 minutes

➲ *CPT Changes: An Insider's View* 2020

➲ *CPT Assistant* Jan 20:3, Mar 20:6

 # 99422 11-20 minutes

➲ *CPT Changes: An Insider's View* 2020

➲ *CPT Assistant* Jan 20:3, Mar 20:6

 # 99423 21 or more minutes

➲ *CPT Changes: An Insider's View* 2020

➲ *CPT Assistant* Jan 20:3, Mar 20:6

(Report 99421, 99422, 99423 once per 7-day period)

(Clinical staff time is not calculated as part of cumulative time for 99421, 99422, 99423)

(Do not report online digital E/M services for cumulative service time less than 5 minutes)

(Do not count 99421, 99422, 99423 time otherwise reported with other services)

►(Do not report 99421, 99422, 99423 on a day when the physician or other qualified health care professional reports E/M services [99202, 99203, 99204, 99205, 99212, 99213, 99214, 99215, 99241, 99242, 99243, 99244, 99245])◄

►(Do not report 99421, 99422, 99423 when using 99091, 99339, 99340, 99374, 99375, 99377, 99378, 99379, 99380, 99487, 99489 for the same communication[s])◄

(Do not report 99421, 99422, 99423 for home and outpatient INR monitoring when reporting 93792, 93793)

(99444 has been deleted. To report, see 99421, 99422, 99423)

Interprofessional Telephone/Internet/Electronic Health Record Consultations

The consultant should use codes 99446, 99447, 99448, 99449, 99451 to report interprofessional telephone/Internet/electronic health record consultations. An interprofessional telephone/Internet/electronic health record consultation is an assessment and management service in which a patient's treating (eg, attending or primary) physician or other qualified health care professional requests the opinion and/or treatment advice of a physician with specific specialty expertise (the consultant) to assist the treating physician or other qualified health care professional in the diagnosis and/or management of the patient's problem without patient face-to-face contact with the consultant.

The patient for whom the interprofessional telephone/Internet/electronic health record consultation is requested may be either a new patient to the consultant or an established patient with a new problem or an exacerbation of an existing problem. However, the consultant should not have seen the patient in a face-to-face encounter within the last 14 days. When the telephone/Internet/electronic health record consultation leads to a transfer of care or other face-to-face service (eg, a surgery, a hospital visit, or a scheduled office evaluation of the patient) within the next 14 days or next available appointment date of the consultant, these codes are not reported.

Review of pertinent medical records, laboratory studies, imaging studies, medication profile, pathology specimens, etc is included in the telephone/Internet/electronic health record consultation service and should not be reported separately when reporting 99446, 99447, 99448, 99449, 99451. The majority of the service time reported (greater than 50%) must be devoted to the medical consultative verbal or Internet discussion. If greater than 50% of the time for the service is devoted to data review and/or analysis, 99446, 99447, 99448, 99449 should not be reported. However, the service time for 99451 is based on total review and interprofessional-communication time.

If more than one telephone/Internet/electronic health record contact(s) is required to complete the consultation request (eg, discussion of test results), the entirety of the service and the cumulative discussion and information review time should be reported with a single code. Codes 99446, 99447, 99448, 99449, 99451 should not be reported more than once within a seven-day interval.

The written or verbal request for telephone/Internet/electronic health record advice by the treating/requesting physician or other qualified health care professional should be documented in the patient's medical record, including the reason for the request. Codes 99446, 99447, 99448, 99449 conclude with a verbal opinion report and written report from the consultant to the treating/requesting physician or other qualified health care professional. Code 99451 concludes with only a written report.

Telephone/Internet/electronic health record consultations of less than five minutes should not be reported. Consultant communications with the patient and/or family may be reported using 98966, 98967, 98968, 99421, 99422, 99423, 99441, 99442, 99443, and the time related to these services is not used in reporting 99446, 99447, 99448, 99449. Do not report 99358, 99359 for any time within the service period, if reporting 99446, 99447, 99448, 99449, 99451.

When the sole purpose of the telephone/Internet/electronic health record communication is to arrange a transfer of care or other face-to-face service, these codes are not reported.

The treating/requesting physician or other qualified health care professional may report 99452 if spending 16-30 minutes in a service day preparing for the referral and/or communicating with the consultant. Do not report 99452 more than once in a 14-day period. The treating/requesting physician or other qualified health care professional may report the prolonged service codes 99354, 99355, 99356, 99357 for the time spent on the interprofessional telephone/Internet/electronic health record discussion with the consultant (eg, specialist) if the time **exceeds 30 minutes** beyond the typical time of the appropriate E/M service performed and the patient is present (on-site) and accessible to the treating/requesting physician or other qualified health care professional. If the interprofessional telephone/Internet/electronic health record assessment and management service occurs when the patient is not present and the time spent in a day **exceeds 30 minutes,** then the non-face-to-face prolonged service codes 99358, 99359 may be reported by the treating/requesting physician or other qualified health care professional.

(For telephone services provided by a physician to a patient, see 99441, 99442, 99443)

(For telephone services provided by a qualified health care professional to a patient, see 98966, 98967, 98968)

(For online digital E/M services provided by a physician or other qualified health care professional to a patient, see 99421, 99422, 99423)

99446 Interprofessional telephone/Internet/electronic health record assessment and management service provided by a consultative physician, including a verbal and written report to the patient's treating/requesting physician or other qualified health care professional; 5-10 minutes of medical consultative discussion and review

➲ *CPT Changes: An Insider's View* 2014, 2019

➲ *CPT Assistant* Jun 14:14, Jan 19:3, Jun 19:7

99447 11-20 minutes of medical consultative discussion and review

➲ *CPT Changes: An Insider's View* 2014, 2019

➲ *CPT Assistant* Jun 14:14, Jan 19:3, Jun 19:7

99448 21-30 minutes of medical consultative discussion and review

➲ *CPT Changes: An Insider's View* 2014, 2019

➲ *CPT Assistant* Jun 14:14, Jan 19:3, Jun 19:7

99449 31 minutes or more of medical consultative discussion and review

➲ *CPT Changes: An Insider's View* 2014, 2019

➲ *CPT Assistant* Jun 14:14, Jan 19:3, Jun 19:7

 # 99451 Interprofessional telephone/Internet/electronic health record assessment and management service provided by a consultative physician, including a written report to the patient's treating/requesting physician or other qualified health care professional, 5 minutes or more of medical consultative time

➲ *CPT Changes: An Insider's View* 2019

➲ *CPT Assistant* Jan 19:3, Jun 19:7

 # 99452 Interprofessional telephone/Internet/electronic health record referral service(s) provided by a treating/requesting physician or other qualified health care professional, 30 minutes

➲ *CPT Changes: An Insider's View* 2019

➲ *CPT Assistant* Jan 19:3, Jun 19:7

Digitally Stored Data Services/Remote Physiologic Monitoring

Codes 99453 and 99454 are used to report remote physiologic monitoring services (eg, weight, blood pressure, pulse oximetry) during a 30-day period. To report 99453, 99454, the device used must be a medical device as defined by the FDA, and the service must be ordered by a physician or other qualified health care professional. Code 99453 may be used to report the set-up and patient education on use of the device(s). Code 99454 may be used to report supply of the device for daily recording or programmed alert transmissions. Codes 99453, 99454 are not reported if monitoring is less than 16 days. Do not report 99453, 99454 when these services are included in other codes for the duration of time of the physiologic monitoring service (eg, 95250 for continuous glucose monitoring requires a minimum of 72 hours of monitoring).

Code 99091 should be reported no more than once in a 30-day period to include the physician or other qualified health care professional time involved with data accession, review and interpretation, modification of care plan as necessary (including communication to patient and/or caregiver), and associated documentation.

If the services described by 99091 or 99474 are provided on the same day the patient presents for an evaluation and management (E/M) service to the same provider, these services should be considered part of the E/M service and not reported separately.

►Do not report 99091 for time in the same calendar month when used to meet the criteria for care plan oversight services (99374, 99375, 99377, 99378, 99379, 99380), home, domiciliary, or rest home care plan oversight services (99339, 99340), remote physiologic monitoring services (99457), or personally performed chronic care management (99491). Do not report 99091 if other more specific codes exist (eg, 93227, 93272 for cardiographic services; 95250 for continuous glucose monitoring). Do not report 99091 for transfer and interpretation of data from hospital or clinical laboratory computers.◀

Code 99453 is reported for each episode of care. For coding remote monitoring of physiologic parameters, an episode of care is defined as beginning when the remote monitoring physiologic service is initiated, and ends with attainment of targeted treatment goals.

 # 99453 Remote monitoring of physiologic parameter(s) (eg, weight, blood pressure, pulse oximetry, respiratory flow rate), initial; set-up and patient education on use of equipment

➲ *CPT Changes: An Insider's View* 2019

➲ *CPT Assistant* Jan 19:3, Mar 19:10

(Do not report 99453 more than once per episode of care)

(Do not report 99453 for monitoring of less than 16 days)

 # 99454 device(s) supply with daily recording(s) or programmed alert(s) transmission, each 30 days

➲ *CPT Changes: An Insider's View* 2019

➲ *CPT Assistant* Jan 19:3, Mar 19:10

(For physiologic monitoring treatment management services, use 99457)

(Do not report 99454 for monitoring of less than 16 days)

(Do not report 99453, 99454 in conjunction with codes for more specific physiologic parameters [eg, 93296, 94760])

(For self-measured blood pressure monitoring, see 99473, 99474)

 # 99091 Collection and interpretation of physiologic data (eg, ECG, blood pressure, glucose monitoring) digitally stored and/or transmitted by the patient and/or caregiver to the physician or other qualified health care professional, qualified by education, training, licensure/regulation (when applicable) requiring a minimum of 30 minutes of time, each 30 days

➲ *CPT Changes: An Insider's View* 2002, 2013, 2019

➲ *CPT Assistant* May 02:19, Jun 03:10, Aug 06:6, Sep 06:15, Jan 07:30, Apr 09:7, Dec 09:6, Apr 13:3, Nov 13:3, Oct 14:3, Feb 18:7, Mar 18:5, Dec 18:11, Feb 20:7, Apr 20:5

(Do not report 99091 in conjunction with 99457)

▶(Do not report 99091 for time in a calendar month when used to meet the criteria for 99339, 99340, 99374, 99375, 99377, 99378, 99379, 99380, 99457, 99491)◀

 # 99473 Self-measured blood pressure using a device validated for clinical accuracy; patient education/training and device calibration

➲ *CPT Changes: An Insider's View* 2020

➲ *CPT Assistant* Jan 20:3, Feb 20:7, Apr 20:5

(Do not report 99473 more than once per device)

(For ambulatory blood pressure monitoring, see 93784, 93786, 93788, 93790)

 # 99474 separate self-measurements of two readings one minute apart, twice daily over a 30-day period (minimum of 12 readings), collection of data reported by the patient and/or caregiver to the physician or other qualified health care professional, with report of average systolic and diastolic pressures and subsequent communication of a treatment plan to the patient

➲ *CPT Changes: An Insider's View* 2020

➲ *CPT Assistant* Jan 20:3, Feb 20:7, Apr 20:5

▶(Do not report 99473, 99474 in the same calendar month as 93784, 93786, 93788, 93790, 99091, 99439, 99453, 99454, 99457, 99487, 99489, 99490, 99491)◀

(Do not report 99474 more than once per calendar month)

Remote Physiologic Monitoring Treatment Management Services

►Remote physiologic monitoring treatment management services are provided when clinical staff/physician/other qualified health care professional use the results of remote physiological monitoring to manage a patient under a specific treatment plan. To report remote physiological monitoring, the device used must be a medical device as defined by the FDA, and the service must be ordered by a physician or other qualified health care professional. Do not use 99457, 99458 for time that can be reported using more specific monitoring services (eg, for the patient that requires reevaluation of medication regimen and/or changes in treatment). Codes 99457, 99458 may be reported during the same service period as chronic care management services (99439, 99487, 99489, 99490, 99491), transitional care management services (99495, 99496), and behavioral health integration services (99484, 99492, 99493, 99494); however, time spent performing these services should remain separate and no time should be counted toward the required time for both services in a single month. Codes 99457, 99458 require a live, interactive communication with the patient/caregiver. For the first completed 20 minutes of clinical staff/physician/other qualified health care professional time in a calendar month report 99457, and report 99458 for each additional completed 20 minutes. Do not report 99457, 99458 for services of less than 20 minutes. Report 99457 one time regardless of the number of physiologic monitoring modalities performed in a given calendar month.

Do not count any time on a day when the physician or other qualified health care professional reports an E/M service (office or other outpatient services 99202, 99203, 99204, 99205, 99211, 99212, 99213, 99214, 99215, domiciliary, rest home services 99324, 99325, 99326, 99327, 99328, 99334, 99335, 99336, 99337, home services 99341, 99342, 99343, 99344, 99345, 99347, 99348, 99349, 99350, inpatient services 99221, 99222, 99223, 99231, 99232, 99233, 99251, 99252, 99253, 99254, 99255). Do not count any time related to other reported services (eg, 93290, 93793, 99291, 99292).◄

 # 99457 Remote physiologic monitoring treatment management services, clinical staff/physician/other qualified health care professional time in a calendar month requiring interactive communication with the patient/caregiver during the month; first 20 minutes

➲ *CPT Changes: An Insider's View* 2019, 2020

➲ *CPT Assistant* Jan 19:3, Jun 19:3, Feb 20:7, Apr 20:5

(Report 99457 once each 30 days, regardless of the number of parameters monitored)

(Do not report 99457 for services of less than 20 minutes)

(Do not report 99457 in conjunction with 93264, 99091)

(Do not report 99457 in the same month as 99473, 99474)

#+ 99458 each additional 20 minutes (List separately in addition to code for primary procedure)

➲ *CPT Changes: An Insider's View* 2020

➲ *CPT Assistant* Feb 20:7

(Use 99458 in conjunction with 99457)

(Do not report 99458 for services of less than an additional increment of 20 minutes)

Special Evaluation and Management Services

The following codes are used to report evaluations performed to establish baseline information prior to life or disability insurance certificates being issued. This service is performed in the office or other setting, and applies to both new and established patients. When using these codes, no active management of the problem(s) is undertaken during the encounter.

If other evaluation and management services and/or procedures are performed on the same date, the appropriate E/M or procedure code(s) should be reported in addition to these codes.

Basic Life and/or Disability Evaluation Services

99450 **Basic life** and/or disability examination that includes:

- **Measurement of height, weight, and blood pressure;**
- **Completion of a medical history following a life insurance pro forma;**
- **Collection of blood sample and/or urinalysis complying with "chain of custody" protocols; and**
- **Completion of necessary documentation/certificates.**

CPT Assistant Summer 95:14, Sep 98:5, May 05:1, Jun 19:7

99451 Code is out of numerical sequence. See 99448-99455

99452 Code is out of numerical sequence. See 99448-99455

99453 Code is out of numerical sequence. See 99448-99455

99454 Code is out of numerical sequence. See 99448-99455

Work Related or Medical Disability Evaluation Services

99455 **Work related** or medical disability examination by the treating physician that includes:

- **Completion of a medical history commensurate with the patient's condition;**
- **Performance of an examination commensurate with the patient's condition;**
- **Formulation of a diagnosis, assessment of capabilities and stability, and calculation of impairment;**
- **Development of future medical treatment plan; and**
- **Completion of necessary documentation/certificates and report.**

CPT Assistant Summer 95:14, Sep 98:5, May 05:1, Aug 13:13

99456 **Work related** or medical disability examination by other than the treating physician that includes:

- **Completion of a medical history commensurate with the patient's condition;**
- **Performance of an examination commensurate with the patient's condition;**
- **Formulation of a diagnosis, assessment of capabilities and stability, and calculation of impairment;**
- **Development of future medical treatment plan; and**
- **Completion of necessary documentation/certificates and report.**

CPT Assistant Summer 95:14, Sep 98:5, Aug 13:13

(Do not report 99455, 99456 in conjunction with 99080 for the completion of Workman's Compensation forms)

99457 Code is out of numerical sequence. See 99448-99455

99458 Code is out of numerical sequence. See 99448-99455

Newborn Care Services

The following codes are used to report the services provided to newborns (birth through the first 28 days) in several different settings. Use of the normal newborn codes is limited to the initial care of the newborn in the first days after birth prior to home discharge.

Evaluation and Management (E/M) services for the newborn include maternal and/or fetal and newborn history, newborn physical examination(s), ordering of diagnostic tests and treatments, meetings with the family, and documentation in the medical record.

When delivery room attendance services (99464) or delivery room resuscitation services (99465) are required, report these in addition to normal newborn services Evaluation and Management codes.

For E/M services provided to newborns who are other than normal, see codes for hospital inpatient services (99221-99233) and neonatal intensive and critical care services (99466-99469, 99477-99480). When normal newborn services are provided by the same individual on the same date that the newborn later becomes ill and receives additional intensive or critical care services, report the appropriate E/M code with modifier 25 for these services in addition to the normal newborn code.

Procedures (eg, 54150, newborn circumcision) are not included with the normal newborn codes, and when performed, should be reported in addition to the newborn services.

►When newborns are seen in follow-up after the date of discharge in the office or outpatient setting, see 99202-99215, 99381, 99391 as appropriate.◄

99460 Initial hospital or birthing center care, per day, for evaluation and management of normal newborn infant

➲ *CPT Changes: An Insider's View* 2009

99461 Initial care, per day, for evaluation and management of normal newborn infant seen in other than hospital or birthing center

➲ *CPT Changes: An Insider's View* 2009

99462 Subsequent hospital care, per day, for evaluation and management of normal newborn

➲ *CPT Changes: An Insider's View* 2009

99463 Initial hospital or birthing center care, per day, for evaluation and management of normal newborn infant admitted and discharged on the same date

➲ *CPT Changes: An Insider's View* 2009

(For newborn hospital discharge services provided on a date subsequent to the admission date, see 99238, 99239)

Delivery/Birthing Room Attendance and Resuscitation Services

99464 Attendance at delivery (when requested by the delivering physician or other qualified health care professional) and initial stabilization of newborn

➲ *CPT Changes: An Insider's View* 2009, 2013

(99464 may be reported in conjunction with 99460, 99468, 99477)

(Do not report 99464 in conjunction with 99465)

99465 Delivery/birthing room resuscitation, provision of positive pressure ventilation and/or chest compressions in the presence of acute inadequate ventilation and/or cardiac output

➲ *CPT Changes: An Insider's View* 2009

(99465 may be reported in conjunction with 99460, 99468, 99477)

(Do not report 99465 in conjunction with 99464)

(Procedures that are performed as a necessary part of the resuscitation [eg, intubation, vascular lines] are reported separately in addition to 99465. In order to report these procedures, they must be performed as a necessary component of the resuscitation and not as a convenience before admission to the neonatal intensive care unit)

Inpatient Neonatal Intensive Care Services and Pediatric and Neonatal Critical Care Services

Pediatric Critical Care Patient Transport

Codes 99466, 99467 are used to report the physical attendance and direct face-to-face care by a physician during the interfacility transport of a critically ill or critically injured pediatric patient 24 months of age or younger. Codes 99485, 99486 are used to report the control physician's non-face-to-face supervision of interfacility transport of a critically ill or critically injured pediatric patient 24 months of age or younger. These codes are not reported together for the same patient by the same physician. For the purpose of reporting 99466 and 99467, face-to-face care begins when the physician assumes primary responsibility of the pediatric patient at the referring facility, and ends when the receiving facility accepts responsibility for the pediatric patient's care. Only the time the physician spends in direct face-to-face contact with the patient during the transport should be reported. Pediatric patient transport services involving less than 30 minutes of face-to-face physician care should not be reported using 99466, 99467. Procedure(s) or service(s) performed by other members of the transporting team may not be reported by the supervising physician.

Codes 99485, 99486 may be used to report control physician's non-face-to-face supervision of interfacility pediatric critical care transport, which includes all two-way communication between the control physician and the specialized transport team prior to transport, at the referring facility and during transport of the patient back to the receiving facility. The "control" physician is the physician directing transport services. These codes do not include pretransport communication between the control physician and the referring facility before or following patient transport. These codes may only be reported for patients 24 months of age or younger who are critically ill or critically injured. The control physician provides treatment advice to a specialized transport team who are present and delivering the hands-on patient care. The control physician does not report any services provided by the specialized transport team. The control physician's non-face-to-face time begins with the first contact by the control physician with the specialized transport team and ends when the patient's care is handed over to the receiving facility team. Refer to 99466 and 99467 for face-to-face transport care of the critically ill/injured patient. Time spent with the individual patient's transport team and reviewing data submissions should be recorded. Code 99485 is used to report the first 16-45 minutes of direction on a given date and should only be used once even if time spent by the physician is discontinuous. Do not report services of 15 minutes or less or any time when another physician is reporting 99466, 99467. Do not report 99485 or 99486 in conjunction with 99466, 99467 when performed by the same physician.

For the definition of the critically injured pediatric patient, see the **Neonatal and Pediatric Critical Care Services** section.

The non-face-to-face direction of emergency care to a patient's transporting staff by a physician located in a hospital or other facility by two-way communication is not considered direct face-to-face care and should not be reported with 99466, 99467. Physician-directed non-face-to-face emergency care through outside voice communication to transporting staff personnel is reported with 99288 or 99485, 99486 based upon the age and clinical condition of the patient.

Emergency department services (99281-99285), initial hospital care (99221-99223), critical care (99291, 99292), initial date neonatal intensive (99477) or critical care (99468) may only be reported after the patient has been admitted to the emergency department, the inpatient floor, or the critical care unit of the receiving facility. If inpatient critical care services are reported in the referring facility prior to transfer to the receiving hospital, use the critical care codes (99291, 99292).

The following services are included when performed during the pediatric patient transport by the physician providing critical care and may not be reported separately: routine monitoring evaluations (eg, heart rate, respiratory rate, blood pressure, and pulse oximetry), the interpretation of cardiac output measurements (93562), chest X rays (71045, 71046), pulse oximetry (94760, 94761, 94762), blood gases and information data stored in computers (eg, ECGs, blood pressures, hematologic data), gastric intubation (43752, 43753), temporary transcutaneous pacing (92953), ventilatory management (94002, 94003, 94660, 94662), and vascular access procedures (36000, 36400, 36405, 36406, 36415, 36591, 36600). Any services performed which are not listed above should be reported separately.

Services provided by the specialized transport team during non-face-to-face transport supervision are not reported by the control physician.

Code 99466 is used to report the first 30 to 74 minutes of direct face-to-face time with the transport pediatric patient and should be reported only once on a given date. Code 99467 is used to report each additional 30 minutes provided on a given date. Face-to-face services of less than 30 minutes should not be reported with these codes.

Code 99485 is used to report the first 30 minutes of non-face-to-face supervision of an interfacility transport of a critically ill or critically injured pediatric patient and should be reported only once per date of service. Only the communication time spent by the supervising physician with the specialty transport team members during an interfacility transport should be reported. Code 99486 is used to report each additional 30 minutes beyond the initial 30 minutes. Non-face-to-face interfacility transport of 15 minutes or less is not reported.

(For total body and selective head cooling of neonates, use 99184)

99466 **Critical care** face-to-face services, during an interfacility transport of critically ill or critically injured pediatric patient, 24 months of age or younger; first 30-74 minutes of hands-on care during transport

➔ *CPT Changes: An Insider's View* 2009, 2013

➔ *CPT Assistant* Sep 11:3, May 13:6, May 14:4, Jun 18:9

+ 99467 each additional 30 minutes (List separately in addition to code for primary service)

➔ *CPT Changes: An Insider's View* 2009, 2013

➔ *CPT Assistant* Sep 11:3, May 13:6, May 14:4, Jun 18:9

(Use 99467 in conjunction with 99466)

(Critical care of less than 30 minutes total duration should be reported with the appropriate E/M code)

 # 99485 Supervision by a control physician of interfacility transport care of the critically ill or critically injured pediatric patient, 24 months of age or younger, includes two-way communication with transport team before transport, at the referring facility and during the transport, including data interpretation and report; first 30 minutes

➔ *CPT Changes: An Insider's View* 2013

➔ *CPT Assistant* May 13:6, May 14:4, Jun 18:9

#+ 99486 each additional 30 minutes (List separately in addition to code for primary procedure)

➔ *CPT Changes: An Insider's View* 2013

➔ *CPT Assistant* May 13:6, May 14:4, Jun 18:9

(Use 99486 in conjunction with 99485)

(For physician direction of emergency medical systems supervision for a pediatric patient older than 24 months of age, or at any age if not critically ill or injured, use 99288)

(Do not report 99485, 99486 with any other services reported by the control physician for the same period)

(Do not report 99485, 99486 in conjunction with 99466, 99467 when performed by the same physician)

Inpatient Neonatal and Pediatric Critical Care

The same definitions for critical care services apply for the adult, child, and neonate.

Codes 99468, 99469 may be used to report the services of directing the inpatient care of a critically ill neonate or infant 28 days of age or younger. They represent care starting with the date of admission (99468) for critical care services and all subsequent day(s) (99469) that the neonate remains in critical care. These codes may be reported only by a single individual and only once per calendar day, per patient. Initial inpatient neonatal critical care (99468) may only be reported once per hospital admission. If readmitted for neonatal critical care services during the same hospital stay, then report the subsequent inpatient neonatal critical care code (99469) for the first day of readmission to critical care, and 99469 for each day of critical care following readmission.

The initial inpatient neonatal critical care code (99468) can be used in addition to 99464 or 99465 as appropriate, when the physician or other qualified health care professional is present for the delivery (99464) or resuscitation (99465) is required. Other procedures performed as a necessary part of the resuscitation (eg, endotracheal intubation [31500]) may also be reported separately, when performed as part of the pre-admission delivery room care. In order to report these procedures separately, they must be performed as a necessary component of the resuscitation and not simply as a convenience before admission to the neonatal intensive care unit.

Codes 99471-99476 may be used to report the services of directing the inpatient care of a critically ill infant or young child from 29 days of postnatal age through 5 years of age. They represent care starting with the date of admission (99471, 99475) for pediatric critical care services and all subsequent day(s) (99472, 99476) that the infant or child remains in critical condition. These codes may only be reported by a single individual and only once per calendar day, per patient. Services for the critically ill or critically injured child 6 years of age or older would be reported with the time-based critical care codes (99291, 99292). Initial inpatient critical care (99471, 99475) may only be reported once per hospital admission. If readmitted to the pediatric critical care unit during the same hospital stay, then report the subsequent inpatient pediatric critical care code 99472 or 99476 for the first day of readmission to critical care and 99472 or 99476 for each day of critical care following readmission.

The pediatric and neonatal critical care codes include those procedures listed for the critical care codes (99291, 99292). In addition, the following procedures are also included (and are not separately reported by professionals, but may be reported by facilities) in the pediatric and neonatal critical care service codes (99468-99472, 99475, 99476) and the intensive care services codes (99477-99480).

Any services performed that are not included in these listings may be reported separately. For initiation of selective head or total body hypothermia in the critically ill neonate, report 99184. Facilities may report the included services separately.

Invasive or non-invasive electronic monitoring of vital signs

Vascular access procedures

- Peripheral vessel catheterization (36000)
- Other arterial catheters (36140, 36620)
- Umbilical venous catheters (36510)
- Central vessel catheterization (36555)
- Vascular access procedures (36400, 36405, 36406)
- Vascular punctures (36420, 36600)
- Umbilical arterial catheters (36660)

Airway and ventilation management

Endotracheal intubation (31500)

Ventilatory management (94002-94004)

Bedside pulmonary function testing (94375)

Surfactant administration (94610)

Continuous positive airway pressure (CPAP) (94660)

Monitoring or interpretation of blood gases or oxygen saturation (94760-94762)

Car Seat Evaluation (94780-94781)

Transfusion of blood components (36430, 36440)

Oral or nasogastric tube placement (43752)

Suprapubic bladder aspiration (51100)

Bladder catheterization (51701, 51702)

Lumbar puncture (62270)

Any services performed which are not listed above may be reported separately.

When a neonate or infant is not critically ill but requires intensive observation, frequent interventions, and other intensive care services, the Continuing Intensive Care Services codes (99477-99480) should be used to report these services.

To report critical care services provided in the outpatient setting (eg, emergency department or office) for neonates and pediatric patients of any age, see the Critical Care codes 99291, 99292. If the same individual provides critical care services for a neonatal or pediatric patient less than 6 years of age in both the outpatient and inpatient settings on the same day, report only the appropriate Neonatal or Pediatric Critical Care codes 99468-99476 for all critical care services provided on that day. Critical care services provided by a second individual of a different specialty not reporting a per-day neonatal or pediatric critical care code can be reported with 99291, 99292.

When critical care services are provided to neonates or pediatric patients less than 6 years of age at two separate institutions by an individual from a different group on the same date of service, the individual from the referring institution should report their critical care services with the time-based critical care codes (99291, 99292) and the receiving institution should report the appropriate initial day of care code 99468, 99471, 99475 for the same date of service.

Critical care services to a pediatric patient 6 years of age or older are reported with the time based critical care codes 99291, 99292.

When the critically ill neonate or pediatric patient improves and is transferred to a lower level of care to another individual in another group within the same facility, the transferring individual does not report a per day critical care service. Subsequent hospital care (99231-99233) or time-based critical care services (99291-99292) is reported, as appropriate based upon the condition of the neonate or child. The receiving individual reports subsequent intensive care (99478-99480) or subsequent hospital care (99231-99233) services, as appropriate based upon the condition of the neonate or child.

When the neonate or infant becomes critically ill on a day when initial or subsequent intensive care services (99477-99480), hospital services (99221-99233), or normal newborn services (99460, 99461, 99462) have been performed by one individual and is transferred to a critical care level of care provided by a different individual in a different group, the transferring individual reports either the time-based critical care services performed (99291, 99292) for the time spent providing critical care to the patient, the intensive care service (99477-99480), hospital care services (99221-99233), or normal newborn service (99460, 99461, 99462) performed, but only one service. The receiving individual reports initial or subsequent inpatient neonatal or pediatric critical care (99468-99476), as appropriate based upon the patient's age and whether this is the first or subsequent admission to the critical care unit for the hospital stay.

When a newborn becomes critically ill on the same day they have already received normal newborn care (99460, 99461, 99462), and the same individual or group assumes critical care, report initial critical care service (99468) with modifier 25 in addition to the normal newborn code.

When a neonate, infant, or child requires initial critical care services on the same day the patient already has received hospital care or intensive care services by the same individual or group, only the initial critical care service code (99468, 99471, 99475) is reported.

Time-based critical care services (99291, 99292) are not reportable by the same individual or different individual of the same specialty and same group, when neonatal or pediatric critical care services (99468-99476) may be reported for the same patient on the same day. Time-based critical care services (99291, 99292) may be reported by an individual of a different specialty from either the same or different group on the same day that neonatal or pediatric critical care services are reported. Critical care interfacility transport face-to-face (99466, 99467) or supervisory (99485, 99486) services may be reported by the same or different individual of the same specialty and same group, when neonatal or pediatric critical care services (99468-99476) are reported for the same patient on the same day.

99468 **Initial inpatient neonatal critical care,** per day, for the evaluation and management of a critically ill neonate, 28 days of age or younger

CPT Changes: An Insider's View 2009

CPT Assistant Nov 11:5, May 14:4, Feb 15:10, Oct 15:8, May 16:3, Jun 18:9, Dec 18:8

99469 **Subsequent inpatient neonatal critical care,** per day, for the evaluation and management of a critically ill neonate, 28 days of age or younger

CPT Changes: An Insider's View 2009

CPT Assistant Nov 11:5, May 14:4, Feb 15:10, Oct 15:8, May 16:4, Jun 18:9, Dec 18:8

99471 **Initial inpatient pediatric critical care,** per day, for the evaluation and management of a critically ill infant or young child, 29 days through 24 months of age

CPT Changes: An Insider's View 2009

CPT Assistant Nov 11:5, Feb 15:10, May 16:3, Jun 18:9, Dec 18:8

99472 **Subsequent inpatient pediatric critical care,** per day, for the evaluation and management of a critically ill infant or young child, 29 days through 24 months of age

CPT Changes: An Insider's View 2009

CPT Assistant Nov 11:5, Feb 15:10, May 16:4, Jun 18:9, Dec 18:8

99473 Code is out of numerical sequence. See 99448-99455

99474 Code is out of numerical sequence. See 99448-99455

99475 **Initial inpatient pediatric critical care,** per day, for the evaluation and management of a critically ill infant or young child, 2 through 5 years of age

CPT Changes: An Insider's View 2009

CPT Assistant Feb 15:10, May 16:3, Jun 18:9, Dec 18:8

99476 **Subsequent inpatient pediatric critical care,** per day, for the evaluation and management of a critically ill infant or young child, 2 through 5 years of age

CPT Changes: An Insider's View 2009

CPT Assistant Feb 15:10, May 16:4, Jun 18:9, Dec 18:8

Initial and Continuing Intensive Care Services

Code 99477 represents the initial day of inpatient care for the child who is not critically ill but requires intensive observation, frequent interventions, and other intensive care services. Codes 99478-99480 are used to report the subsequent day services of directing

E/M 99202-99499

the continuing intensive care of the low birth weight (LBW 1500-2500 grams) present body weight infant, very low birth weight (VLBW less than 1500 grams) present body weight infant, or normal (2501-5000 grams) present body weight newborn who does not meet the definition of critically ill but continues to require intensive observation, frequent interventions, and other intensive care services. These services are for infants and neonates who are not critically ill but continue to require intensive cardiac and respiratory monitoring, continuous and/or frequent vital sign monitoring, heat maintenance, enteral and/or parenteral nutritional adjustments, laboratory and oxygen monitoring, and constant observation by the health care team under direct supervision of the physician or other qualified health care professional. Codes 99477-99480 may be reported by a single individual and only once per day, per patient in a given facility. If readmitted to the intensive care unit during the same hospital stay, report 99478-99480 for the first day of intensive care and for each successive day that the child requires intensive care services.

These codes include the same procedures that are outlined in the **Neonatal and Pediatric Critical Care Services** section and these services should not be separately reported.

The initial day neonatal intensive care code (99477) can be used in addition to 99464 or 99465 as appropriate, when the physician or other qualified health care professional is present for the delivery (99464) or resuscitation (99465) is required. In this situation, report 99477 with modifier 25. Other procedures performed as a necessary part of the resuscitation (eg, endotracheal intubation [31500]) are also reported separately when performed as part of the pre-admission delivery room care. In order to report these procedures separately, they must be performed as a necessary component of the resuscitation and not simply as a convenience before admission to the neonatal intensive care unit.

The same procedures are included as bundled services with the neonatal intensive care codes as those listed for the neonatal (99468, 99469) and pediatric (99471-99476) critical care codes.

When the neonate or infant improves after the initial day and no longer requires intensive care services and is transferred to a lower level of care, the transferring individual does not report a per day intensive care service. Subsequent hospital care (99231-99233) or subsequent normal newborn care (99460, 99462) is reported as appropriate based upon the condition of the neonate or infant. If the transfer to a lower level of care occurs on the same day as initial intensive care services were provided by the transferring individual, 99477 may be reported.

When the neonate or infant is transferred after the initial day within the same facility to the care of another individual in a different group, both individuals report subsequent hospital care (99231-99233) services. The receiving individual reports subsequent hospital care (99231-99233) or subsequent normal newborn care (99462).

When the neonate or infant becomes critically ill on a day when initial or subsequent intensive care services (99477-99480) have been reported by one individual and is transferred to a critical care level of care provided by a different individual from a different group, the transferring individual reports either the time-based critical care services performed (99291, 99292) for the time spent providing critical care to the patient or the initial or subsequent intensive care (99477-99480) service, but not both. The receiving individual reports initial or subsequent inpatient neonatal or pediatric critical care (99468-99476) based upon the patient's age and whether this is the first or subsequent admission to critical care for the same hospital stay.

When the neonate or infant becomes critically ill on a day when initial or subsequent intensive care services (99477-99480) have been performed by the same individual or group, report only initial or subsequent inpatient neonatal or pediatric critical care

(99468-99476) based upon the patient's age and whether this is the first or subsequent admission to critical care for the same hospital stay.

For the subsequent care of the sick neonate younger than 28 days of age but more than 5000 grams who does not require intensive or critical care services, use codes 99231-99233.

99477 **Initial hospital care,** per day, for the evaluation and management of the neonate, 28 days of age or younger, who requires intensive observation, frequent interventions, and other intensive care services

➲ *CPT Changes: An Insider's View* 2008

➲ *CPT Assistant* Jan 08:8, Jul 08:10, Mar 09:3, Nov 11:5, May 14:4, Dec 18:8

(For the initiation of inpatient care of the normal newborn, use 99460)

(For the initiation of care of the critically ill neonate, use 99468)

(For initiation of inpatient hospital care of the ill neonate not requiring intensive observation, frequent interventions, and other intensive care services, see 99221-99223)

99478 **Subsequent intensive care,** per day, for the evaluation and management of the recovering very low birth weight infant (present body weight less than 1500 grams)

➲ *CPT Changes: An Insider's View* 2009

➲ *CPT Assistant* Jun 18:11, Dec 18:8

99479 **Subsequent intensive care,** per day, for the evaluation and management of the recovering low birth weight infant (present body weight of 1500-2500 grams)

➲ *CPT Changes: An Insider's View* 2009

➲ *CPT Assistant* Jun 18:11, Dec 18:8

99480 **Subsequent intensive care,** per day, for the evaluation and management of the recovering infant (present body weight of 2501-5000 grams)

➲ *CPT Changes: An Insider's View* 2009

➲ *CPT Assistant* May 14:4, Jul 15:3, Jun 18:11, Dec 18:8

Cognitive Assessment and Care Plan Services

Cognitive assessment and care plan services are provided when a comprehensive evaluation of a new or existing patient, who exhibits signs and/or symptoms of cognitive impairment, is required to establish or confirm a diagnosis, etiology and severity for the condition. This service includes a thorough evaluation of medical and psychosocial factors, potentially contributing to increased morbidity. Do not report cognitive assessment and care plan services if any of the required elements are not performed or are deemed unnecessary for the patient's condition. For these services, see the appropriate evaluation and management code. A single physician or other qualified health care professional should not report 99483 more than once every 180 days.

Services for cognitive assessment and care plan include a cognition-relevant history, as well as an assessment of factors that could be contributing to cognitive impairment, including, but not limited to, psychoactive medication, chronic pain syndromes, infection, depression and other brain disease (eg, tumor, stroke, normal pressure hydrocephalus). Medical decision making includes current and likely progression of the disease, assessing the need for referral for rehabilitative, social, legal, financial, or community-based services, meal, transportation, and other personal assistance services.

99483 Assessment of and care planning for a patient with cognitive impairment, requiring an independent historian, in the office or other outpatient, home or domiciliary or rest home, with all of the following required elements:

- Cognition-focused evaluation including a pertinent history and examination;
- Medical decision making of moderate or high complexity;
- Functional assessment (eg, basic and instrumental activities of daily living), including decision-making capacity;
- Use of standardized instruments for staging of dementia (eg, functional assessment staging test [FAST], clinical dementia rating [CDR]);
- Medication reconciliation and review for high-risk medications;
- Evaluation for neuropsychiatric and behavioral symptoms, including depression, including use of standardized screening instrument(s);
- Evaluation of safety (eg, home), including motor vehicle operation;
- Identification of caregiver(s), caregiver knowledge, caregiver needs, social supports, and the willingness of caregiver to take on caregiving tasks;
- Development, updating or revision, or review of an Advance Care Plan;
- Creation of a written care plan, including initial plans to address any neuropsychiatric symptoms, neuro-cognitive symptoms, functional limitations, and referral to community resources as needed (eg, rehabilitation services, adult day programs, support groups) shared with the patient and/or caregiver with initial education and support.

Typically, 50 minutes are spent face-to-face with the patient and/or family or caregiver.

➔ *CPT Changes: An Insider's View* 2018

➔ *CPT Assistant* Apr 18:9, Jul 18:12

►(Do not report 99483 in conjunction with E/M services [99202, 99203, 99204, 99205, 99211, 99212, 99213, 99214, 99215, 99241, 99242, 99243, 99244, 99245, 99324, 99325, 99326, 99327, 99328, 99334, 99335, 99336, 99337, 99341, 99342, 99343, 99344, 99345, 99347, 99348, 99349, 99350, 99366, 99367, 99368, 99497, 99498]; psychiatric diagnostic procedures [90785, 90791, 90792]; brief emotional/behavioral assessment [96127]; psychological or neuropsychological test administration [96146]; health risk assessment administration [96160, 96161]; medication therapy management services [99605, 99606, 99607])◄

99484 Code is out of numerical sequence. See 99497-99499

99485 Code is out of numerical sequence. See 99466-99469

99486 Code is out of numerical sequence. See 99466-99469

Care Management Services

Care management services are management and support services provided by clinical staff, under the direction of a physician or other qualified health care professional, or may be provided personally by a physician or other qualified health care professional to a patient residing at home or in a domiciliary, rest home, or assisted living facility. Services include establishing, implementing, revising, or monitoring the care plan, coordinating the care of other professionals and agencies, and educating the patient or caregiver about the patient's condition, care plan, and prognosis. The physician or other qualified health care professional provides or oversees the management and/or coordination of services, as needed, for all medical conditions, psychosocial needs, and activities of daily living.

►A comprehensive plan of care for health problems is based on a physical, mental, cognitive, social, functional, and environmental evaluation. It is intended to provide a simple and concise overview of the patient, and be a useful resource for patients, caregivers, health care professionals, and others, as necessary.

A typical plan of care is not limited to, but may include:

- Problem list
- Expected outcome and prognosis
- Measurable treatment goals
- Cognitive assessment
- Functional assessment
- Symptom management
- Planned interventions
- Medical management
- Environmental evaluation
- Caregiver assessment
- Interaction and coordination with outside resources and other health care professionals and others, as necessary
- Summary of advance directives

The above elements are intended to be a guide for creating a meaningful plan of care rather than a strict set of requirements, so should be addressed only as appropriate for the individual.

The plan of care should include specific and achievable goals for each condition and be relevant to the patient's well-being and lifestyle. When possible, the treatment goals should also be measurable and time bound. The plan should be updated periodically based on status or goal changes. The entire care plan should be reviewed at least annually.

An electronic and/or printed plan of care must be documented and shared with the patient and/or caregiver.

Codes 99487, 99489, 99490, 99491 are reported only once per calendar month and 99439 is reported no more than twice per calendar month. Codes 99439, 99487, 99489, 99490, 99491 may only be reported by the single physician or other qualified health care professional who assumes the care management role with a particular patient for the calendar month.

For 99439, 99487, 99489, 99490 the face-to-face and non-face-to-face time spent by the clinical staff in communicating with the patient and/or family, caregivers, other professionals, and agencies; creating, revising, documenting, and implementing the care plan; or teaching self-management is used in determining the care management clinical staff time for the month. Only the time of the clinical staff of the reporting professional is counted. Only count the time of one clinical staff member when two or more clinical staff members are meeting about the patient. For 99491, only count the time personally spent by the physician or other qualified health care professional. Do not count any of the clinical staff time spent on the day of an initiating visit (the creation of the care plan, initial explanation to the patient and/or caregiver, and obtaining consent).◀

Care management activities performed by clinical staff, or personally by the physician or other qualified health care professional, typically include:

- communication and engagement with patient, family members, guardian or caretaker, surrogate decision makers, and/or other professionals regarding aspects of care;
- communication with home health agencies and other community services utilized by the patient;
- collection of health outcomes data and registry documentation;
- patient and/or family/caregiver education to support self-management, independent living, and activities of daily living;
- assessment and support for treatment regimen adherence and medication management;

- identification of available community and health resources;
- facilitating access to care and services needed by the patient and/or family;
- management of care transitions not reported as part of transitional care management (99495, 99496);
- ongoing review of patient status, including review of laboratory and other studies not reported as part of an E/M service, noted above;
- development, communication, and maintenance of a comprehensive care plan.

►The care management office/practice must have the following capabilities:

- provide 24/7 access to physicians or other qualified health care professionals or clinical staff including providing patients/caregivers with a means to make contact with health care professionals in the practice to address urgent needs regardless of the time of day or day of week;
- provide continuity of care with a designated member of the care team with whom the patient is able to schedule successive routine appointments;
- provide timely access and management for follow-up after an emergency department visit or facility discharge;
- utilize an electronic health record system so that care providers have timely access to clinical information;
- use a standardized methodology to identify patients who require care management services;
- have an internal care management process/function whereby a patient identified as meeting the requirements for these services starts receiving them in a timely manner;
- use a form and format in the medical record that is standardized within the practice;
- be able to engage and educate patients and caregivers as well as coordinate care among all service professionals, as appropriate for each patient;
- reporting physician or other qualified health care professional oversees activities of the care team;
- all care team members providing services are clinically integrated.

Each minute of service time is counted toward only one service. Do not count any time and activities used to meet criteria for another reported service. However, time of clinical staff and time of a physician or other qualified health care professional are distinct when each provides a distinct, separately reportable service to the same patient during the same period of time (eg, calendar month). A list of services not reported in the same calendar month as 99439, 99487, 99489, 99490 is provided in the parenthetical instructions following 99439, 99489. See the parenthetical instruction below 99491 for a list of services not separately reported in the same calendar month that 99491 is reported. Do not report 99439, 99487, 99489, 99490 when reporting 99491 for the same calendar month. If the care management services are performed within the postoperative period of a reported surgery, the same individual may not report 99439, 99487, 99489, 99490, 99491. For service time used for reporting 99439, 99487, 99489, 99490, 99491, do not also include service time used to report 99421, 99422, 99423.

Care management may be reported in any calendar month during which the clinical staff time or physician or other qualified health care professional personal time requirements are met.◄

When behavioral or psychiatric collaborative care management services are also provided, 99484, 99492, 99493, 99494 may be reported in addition.

Chronic Care Management Services

►Chronic care management services are provided when medical and/or psychosocial needs of the patient require establishing, implementing, revising, or monitoring the care plan. Patients who receive chronic care management services have two or more chronic continuous or episodic health conditions that are expected to last at least 12 months, or until the death of the patient, and that place the patient at significant risk of death, acute exacerbation/decompensation, or functional decline. Code 99490 is reported when, during the calendar month, at least 20 minutes of clinical staff time is spent in care management activities. Code 99439 is reported in conjunction with 99490 for each additional 20 minutes of clinical staff time spent in care management activities during the calendar month up to a maximum of 60 minutes total time (ie, 99439 may only be reported twice per calendar month). Code 99491 is reported when 30 minutes of physician or other qualified health care professional personal time is spent in care management activities. Do not report 99439, 99490 in the same calendar month as 99491. If reporting 99491, do not count any physician or other qualified health care professional time on the date of a face-to-face E/M encounter towards the time used in reporting 99491.◄

#▲ 99490 Chronic care management services with the following required elements:

- multiple (two or more) chronic conditions expected to last at least 12 months, or until the death of the patient,
- chronic conditions place the patient at significant risk of death, acute exacerbation/decompensation, or functional decline,
- comprehensive care plan established, implemented, revised, or monitored;

first 20 minutes of clinical staff time directed by a physician or other qualified health care professional, per calendar month.

➲ *CPT Changes: An Insider's View* 2015, 2021

➲ *CPT Assistant* Oct 14:3, Feb 15:3, Feb 18:7, Mar 18:5, Oct 18:9, Feb 20:7

#+● 99439 each additional 20 minutes of clinical staff time directed by a physician or other qualified health care professional, per calendar month (List separately in addition to code for primary procedure)

➲ *CPT Changes: An Insider's View* 2021

►(Use 99439 in conjunction with 99490)◄

(Chronic care management services of less than 20 minutes duration, in a calendar month, are not reported separately)

►(Chronic care management services of 60 minutes or more and requiring moderate or high complexity medical decision making may be reported using 99487, 99489)◄

►(Do not report 99439 more than twice per calendar month)◄

►(Do not report 99439, 99490 in the same calendar month with 90951-90970, 99339, 99340, 99374, 99375, 99377, 99378, 99379, 99380, 99487, 99489, 99491, 99605, 99606, 99607)◄

►(Do not report 99439, 99490 for service time reported with 93792, 93793, 98960, 98961, 98962, 98966, 98967, 98968, 98970, 98971, 98972, 99071, 99078, 99080, 99091, 99358, 99359, 99366, 99367, 99368, 99421, 99422, 99423, 99441, 99442, 99443, 99605, 99606, 99607)◄

►Total Duration of Staff Care Management Services	Chronic Care Management
less than 20 minutes	Not reported separately
20 to 39 minutes	99490 X 1
40-59 minutes	99490 X 1 and 99439 X 1
60 minutes or more (1 hour or more)	99490 X 1 and 99439 X 2 (see also 99487)◄

E/M 99202-99499

 # 99491 Chronic care management services, provided personally by a physician or other qualified health care professional, at least 30 minutes of physician or other qualified health care professional time, per calendar month, with the following required elements:

- multiple (two or more) chronic conditions expected to last at least 12 months, or until the death of the patient;
- chronic conditions place the patient at significant risk of death, acute exacerbation/decompensation, or functional decline;
- comprehensive care plan established, implemented, revised, or monitored.

➲ *CPT Changes: An Insider's View* 2019

➲ *CPT Assistant* Oct 18:9

►(Do not report 99491 in the same calendar month with 90951-90970, 99339, 99340, 99374, 99375, 99377, 99378, 99379, 99380, 99439, 99487, 99489, 99490, 99605, 99606, 99607)◄

►(Do not report 99491 for service time reported with 93792, 93793, 98960, 98961, 98962, 98966, 98967, 98968, 99071, 99078, 99080, 99091, 99358, 99359, 99366, 99367, 99368, 99421, 99422, 99423, 99441, 99442, 99443)◄

►(Do not report 99491 when performed during the service time of 99495, 99496, if reporting 99495, 99496)◄

Complex Chronic Care Management Services

►Complex chronic care management services are provided during a calendar month that includes criteria for chronic care management services including establishing, revising, implementing, or monitoring the care plan; medical, functional, and/or psychosocial problems requiring medical decision making of moderate or high complexity; and clinical staff care management services for at least 60 minutes, under the direction of a physician or other qualified health care professional. Medical decision making as defined in the Evaluation and Management (E/M) guidelines is determined by the problems addressed by the reporting individual during the month.◄

Patients who require complex chronic care management services may be identified by practice-specific or other published algorithms that recognize multiple illnesses, multiple medication use, inability to perform activities of daily living, requirement for a caregiver, and/or repeat admissions or emergency department visits. Typical adult patients who receive complex chronic care management services are treated with three or more prescription medications and may be receiving other types of therapeutic interventions (eg, physical therapy, occupational therapy). Typical pediatric patients receive three or more therapeutic interventions (eg, medications, nutritional support, respiratory therapy). All patients have two or more chronic continuous or episodic health conditions that are expected to last at least 12 months, or until the death of the patient, and that place the patient at significant risk of death, acute exacerbation/decompensation, or functional decline. Typical patients have complex diseases and morbidities and, as a result, demonstrate one or more of the following:

- need for the coordination of a number of specialties and services;
- inability to perform activities of daily living and/or cognitive impairment resulting in poor adherence to the treatment plan without substantial assistance from a caregiver;
- psychiatric and other medical comorbidities (eg, dementia and chronic obstructive pulmonary disease or substance abuse and diabetes) that complicate their care; and/or
- social support requirements or difficulty with access to care.

Total Duration of Staff Care Management Services	Complex Chronic Care Management
less than 60 minutes	Not reported separately
60 to 89 minutes (1 hour - 1 hr. 29 min.)	99487 X 1
90 - 119 minutes (1 hr. 30 min. - 1 hr. 59 min.)	99487 X 1 and 99489 X 1
120 minutes or more (2 hours or more)	99487 X 1 and 99489 X 2 and 99489 for each additional 30 minutes

▲ **99487** Complex chronic care management services with the following required elements:

- multiple (two or more) chronic conditions expected to last at least 12 months, or until the death of the patient,
- chronic conditions place the patient at significant risk of death, acute exacerbation/decompensation, or functional decline,
- comprehensive care plan established, implemented, revised, or monitored,
- moderate or high complexity medical decision making;

first 60 minutes of clinical staff time directed by a physician or other qualified health care professional, per calendar month.

➲ *CPT Changes: An Insider's View* 2013, 2015, 2021

➲ *CPT Assistant* Apr 13:3, Sep 13:15, Nov 13:3, Feb 14:3, Jun 14:3, 5, Oct 14:3, Apr 17:9, Feb 18:7, Mar 18:5, Oct 18:9, Feb 20:7

(Complex chronic care management services of less than 60 minutes duration, in a calendar month, are not reported separately)

+▲ **99489** each additional 30 minutes of clinical staff time directed by a physician or other qualified health care professional, per calendar month (List separately in addition to code for primary procedure)

➲ *CPT Changes: An Insider's View* 2013, 2015, 2021

➲ *CPT Assistant* Apr 13:3, Sep 13:15, Nov 13:3, Jun 14:5, Oct 14:3, Apr 17:9, Feb 18:7, Mar 18:5, Oct 18:9, Feb 20:7

(Report 99489 in conjunction with 99487)

(Do not report 99489 for care management services of less than 30 minutes additional to the first 60 minutes of complex chronic care management services during a calendar month)

►(Do not report 99487, 99489 during the same calendar month with 90951-90970, 99339, 99340, 99374, 99375, 99377, 99378, 99379, 99380, 99439, 99490, 99491, 99605, 99606, 99607)◄

►(Do not report 99487, 99489 for service time reported with 93792, 93793, 98960, 98961, 98962, 98966, 98967, 98968, 98970, 98971, 98972, 99071, 99078, 99080, 99091, 99358, 99359, 99366, 99367, 99368, 99421, 99422, 99423, 99441, 99442, 99443, 99605, 99606, 99607)◄

Coding Tip

If the physician personally performs the clinical staff activities, his or her time may be counted toward the required clinical staff time to meet the elements of the code.

99490 Code is out of numerical sequence. See 99480-99489

99491 Code is out of numerical sequence. See 99480-99489

E/M 99202-99499

Psychiatric Collaborative Care Management Services

Psychiatric collaborative care services are provided under the direction of a treating physician or other qualified health care professional (see definitions below) during a calendar month. These services are reported by the treating physician or other qualified health care professional and include the services of the treating physician or other qualified health care professional, the behavioral health care manager (see definition below), and the psychiatric consultant (see definition below), who has contracted directly with the treating physician or other qualified health care professional, to provide consultation. Patients directed to the behavioral health care manager typically have behavioral health signs and/or symptoms or a newly diagnosed behavioral health condition, may need help in engaging in treatment, have not responded to standard care delivered in a nonpsychiatric setting, or require further assessment and engagement, prior to consideration of referral to a psychiatric care setting.

These services are provided when a patient requires a behavioral health care assessment; establishing, implementing, revising, or monitoring a care plan; and provision of brief interventions.

The following definitions apply to this section:

Definitions

Episode of care patients are treated for an episode of care, which is defined as beginning when the patient is directed by the treating physician or other qualified health care professional to the behavioral health care manager and ending with:

- the attainment of targeted treatment goals, which typically results in the discontinuation of care management services and continuation of usual follow-up with the treating physician or other qualified health care professional; or
- failure to attain targeted treatment goals culminating in referral to a psychiatric care provider for ongoing treatment of the behavioral health condition; or
- lack of continued engagement with no psychiatric collaborative care management services provided over a consecutive six month calendar period (break in episode).

A new episode of care starts after a break in episode of six calendar months or more.

Health care professionals refers to the treating physician or other qualified health care professional who directs the behavioral health care manager and continues to oversee the patient's care, including prescribing medications, providing treatments for medical conditions, and making referrals to specialty care when needed. Evaluation and management (E/M) and other services may be reported separately by the same physician or other qualified health care professional during the same calendar month.

Behavioral health care manager refers to clinical staff with a masters-/doctoral-level education or specialized training in behavioral health who provides care management services as well as an assessment of needs, including the administration of validated rating scales, the development of a care plan, provision of brief interventions, ongoing collaboration with the treating physician or other qualified health care professional, maintenance of a registry, all in consultation with a psychiatric consultant. Services are provided both face-to-face and non-face-to-face and psychiatric consultation is provided minimally on a weekly basis, typically non-face-to-face.

The behavioral health care manager providing other services in the same calendar month, such as psychiatric evaluation (90791, 90792), psychotherapy (90832, 90833, 90834, 90836, 90837, 90838), psychotherapy for crisis (90839, 90840), family psychotherapy (90846, 90847), multiple family group psychotherapy (90849), group psychotherapy (90853), smoking and tobacco use cessation counseling (99406, 99407), and alcohol and/or substance abuse structured screening and brief intervention services

(99408, 99409), may report these services separately. Activities for services reported separately are not included in the time applied to 99492, 99493, 99494.

Type of Service	Total Duration of Collaborative Care Management Over Calendar Month	Code(s)
Initial - 70 minutes	Less than 36 minutes	Not reported separately
	36-85 minutes (36 minutes - 1 hr. 25 minutes)	99492 X 1
Initial plus each additional increment up to 30 minutes	86-115 minutes (1 hr. 26 minutes - 1 hr. 55 minutes)	99492 X 1 AND 99494 X 1
Subsequent - 60 minutes	Less than 31 minutes	Not reported separately
	31-75 minutes (31 minutes - 1 hr. 15 minutes)	99493 X 1
Subsequent plus each additional increment up to 30 minutes	76-105 minutes (1 hr. 16 minutes - 1 hr. 45 minutes)	99493 X 1 AND 99494 X 1

Psychiatric consultant refers to a medical professional, who is trained in psychiatry or behavioral health, and qualified to prescribe the full range of medications. The psychiatric consultant advises and makes recommendations, as needed, for psychiatric and other medical care, including psychiatric and other medical differential diagnosis, treatment strategies regarding appropriate therapies, medication management, medical management of complications associated with treatment of psychiatric disorders, and referral for specialty services, which are typically communicated to the treating physician or other qualified health care professional through the behavioral health care manager. The psychiatric consultant typically does not see the patient or prescribe medications, except in rare circumstances.

The psychiatric consultant may provide services in the calendar month described by other codes, such as evaluation and management (E/M) services and psychiatric evaluation (90791, 90792). These services may be reported separately by the psychiatric consultant. Activities for services reported separately are not included in the services reported using 99492, 99493, 99494.

Do not report 99492 and 99493 in the same calendar month.

99492 **Initial psychiatric collaborative care management,** first 70 minutes in the first calendar month of behavioral health care manager activities, in consultation with a psychiatric consultant, and directed by the treating physician or other qualified health care professional, with the following required elements:

- outreach to and engagement in treatment of a patient directed by the treating physician or other qualified health care professional;
- initial assessment of the patient, including administration of validated rating scales, with the development of an individualized treatment plan;
- review by the psychiatric consultant with modifications of the plan if recommended;
- entering patient in a registry and tracking patient follow-up and progress using the registry, with appropriate documentation, and participation in weekly caseload consultation with the psychiatric consultant; and
- provision of brief interventions using evidence-based techniques such as behavioral activation, motivational interviewing, and other focused treatment strategies.

➔ *CPT Changes: An Insider's View* 2018

➔ *CPT Assistant* Nov 17:3, Feb 18:7, Mar 18:5, Jul 18:12, Feb 20:7

E/M 99202-99499

99493 **Subsequent psychiatric collaborative care management,** first 60 minutes in a subsequent month of behavioral health care manager activities, in consultation with a psychiatric consultant, and directed by the treating physician or other qualified health care professional, with the following required elements:

- tracking patient follow-up and progress using the registry, with appropriate documentation;
- participation in weekly caseload consultation with the psychiatric consultant;
- ongoing collaboration with and coordination of the patient's mental health care with the treating physician or other qualified health care professional and any other treating mental health providers;
- additional review of progress and recommendations for changes in treatment, as indicated, including medications, based on recommendations provided by the psychiatric consultant;
- provision of brief interventions using evidence-based techniques such as behavioral activation, motivational interviewing, and other focused treatment strategies;
- monitoring of patient outcomes using validated rating scales; and
- relapse prevention planning with patients as they achieve remission of symptoms and/or other treatment goals and are prepared for discharge from active treatment.

➲ *CPT Changes: An Insider's View* 2018

➲ *CPT Assistant* Nov 17:3, Feb 18:7, Mar 18:5, Jul 18:12, Feb 20:7

+ 99494 **Initial or subsequent psychiatric collaborative care management,** each additional 30 minutes in a calendar month of behavioral health care manager activities, in consultation with a psychiatric consultant, and directed by the treating physician or other qualified health care professional (List separately in addition to code for primary procedure)

➲ *CPT Changes: An Insider's View* 2018

➲ *CPT Assistant* Nov 17:3, Feb 18:7, Mar 18:5, Jul 18:12, Feb 20:7

(Use 99494 in conjunction with 99492, 99493)

Coding Tip

If the treating physician or other qualified health care professional personally performs behavioral health care manager activities and those activities are not used to meet criteria for a separately reported code, his or her time may be counted toward the required behavioral health care manager time to meet the elements of 99492, 99493, 99494.

Transitional Care Management Services

Codes 99495 and 99496 are used to report transitional care management services (TCM). These services are for a new or established patient whose medical and/or psychosocial problems require moderate or high complexity medical decision making during transitions in care from an inpatient hospital setting (including acute hospital, rehabilitation hospital, long-term acute care hospital), partial hospital, observation status in a hospital, or skilled nursing facility/nursing facility to the patient's community setting (home, domiciliary, rest home, or assisted living). TCM commences upon the date of discharge and continues for the next 29 days.

TCM is comprised of one face-to-face visit within the specified timeframes, in combination with non-face-to-face services that may be performed by the physician or other qualified health care professional and/or licensed clinical staff under his/her direction.

Non-face-to-face services provided by clinical staff, under the direction of the physician or other qualified health care professional, may include:

- communication (with patient, family members, guardian or caretaker, surrogate decision makers, and/or other professionals) regarding aspects of care,

- communication with home health agencies and other community services utilized by the patient,
- patient and/or family/caretaker education to support self-management, independent living, and activities of daily living,
- assessment and support for treatment regimen adherence and medication management,
- identification of available community and health resources,
- facilitating access to care and services needed by the patient and/or family

Non-face-to-face services provided by the physician or other qualified health care provider may include:

- obtaining and reviewing the discharge information (eg, discharge summary, as available, or continuity of care documents);
- reviewing need for or follow-up on pending diagnostic tests and treatments;
- interaction with other qualified health care professionals who will assume or reassume care of the patient's system-specific problems;
- education of patient, family, guardian, and/or caregiver;
- establishment or reestablishment of referrals and arranging for needed community resources;
- assistance in scheduling any required follow-up with community providers and services.

TCM requires a face-to-face visit, initial patient contact, and medication reconciliation within specified time frames. The first face-to-face visit is part of the TCM service and not reported separately. Additional E/M services provided on subsequent dates after the first face-to-face visit may be reported separately. TCM requires an interactive contact with the patient or caregiver, as appropriate, within two business days of discharge. The contact may be direct (face-to-face), telephonic, or by electronic means. Medication reconciliation and management must occur no later than the date of the face-to-face visit.

These services address any needed coordination of care performed by multiple disciplines and community service agencies. The reporting individual provides or oversees the management and/or coordination of services, as needed, for all medical conditions, psychosocial needs and activity of daily living support by providing first contact and continuous access.

Medical decision making and the date of the first face-to-face visit are used to select and report the appropriate TCM code. For 99496, the face-to-face visit must occur within 7 calendar days of the date discharge and medical decision making must be of high complexity. For 99495, the face-to-face visit must occur within 14 calendar days of the date of discharge and medical decision making must be of at least moderate complexity.

Type of Medical Decision Making	Face-to-Face Visit Within 7 Days	Face-to-Face Visit Within 8 to 14 Days
Moderate Complexity	99495	99495
High Complexity	99496	99495

Medical decision making is defined by the E/M Services Guidelines. The medical decision making over the service period reported is used to define the medical decision making of TCM. Documentation includes the timing of the initial post discharge communication with the patient or caregivers, date of the face-to-face visit, and the complexity of medical decision making.

Only one individual may report these services and only once per patient within 30 days of discharge. Another TCM may not be reported by the same individual or group for any

E/M 99202-99499

subsequent discharge(s) within the 30 days. The same individual may report hospital or observation discharge services and TCM. However, the discharge service may not constitute the required face-to-face visit. The same individual should not report TCM services provided in the postoperative period of a service that the individual reported.

★ **99495** **Transitional Care Management Services** with the following required elements:

- Communication (direct contact, telephone, electronic) with the patient and/or caregiver within 2 business days of discharge
- Medical decision making of at least moderate complexity during the service period
- Face-to-face visit, within 14 calendar days of discharge

➲ *CPT Changes: An Insider's View* 2013, 2017

➲ *CPT Assistant* Apr 13:3, Jul 13:11, Aug 13:13, Sep 13:15, Nov 13:3, Dec 13:11, Mar 14:13, Oct 14:3, Feb 18:7, Mar 18:5, Jan 20:3, Feb 20:7

★ **99496** **Transitional Care Management Services** with the following required elements:

- Communication (direct contact, telephone, electronic) with the patient and/or caregiver within 2 business days of discharge
- Medical decision making of high complexity during the service period
- Face-to-face visit, within 7 calendar days of discharge

➲ *CPT Changes: An Insider's View* 2013, 2017

➲ *CPT Assistant* Apr 13:3, Jul 13:11, Aug 13:13, Sep 13:15, Nov 13:3, Mar 14:13, Oct 14:3, Feb 18:7, Mar 18:5, Jan 20:3, Feb 20:7

Coding Tip

If another individual provides TCM services within the postoperative period of a surgical package, modifier 54 is not required.
The required contact with the patient or caregiver, as appropriate, may be by the physician or qualified health care professional or clinical staff. Within two business days of discharge is Monday through Friday except holidays without respect to normal practice hours or date of notification of discharge. The contact must include capacity for prompt interactive communication addressing patient status and needs beyond scheduling follow-up care. If two or more separate attempts are made in a timely manner, but are unsuccessful and other transitional care management criteria are met, the service may be reported.

Advance Care Planning

Codes 99497, 99498 are used to report the face-to-face service between a physician or other qualified health care professional and a patient, family member, or surrogate in counseling and discussing advance directives, with or without completing relevant legal forms. An advance directive is a document appointing an agent and/or recording the wishes of a patient pertaining to his/her medical treatment at a future time should he/she lack decisional capacity at that time. Examples of written advance directives include, but are not limited to, Health Care Proxy, Durable Power of Attorney for Health Care, Living Will, and Medical Orders for Life-Sustaining Treatment (MOLST).

When using codes 99497, 99498, no active management of the problem(s) is undertaken during the time period reported.

▶Codes 99497, 99498 may be reported separately if these services are performed on the same day as another Evaluation and Management service (99202-99215, 99217, 99218, 99219, 99220, 99221, 99222, 99223, 99224, 99225, 99226, 99231, 99232, 99233, 99234, 99235, 99236, 99238, 99239, 99241, 99242, 99243, 99244, 99245, 99251, 99252, 99253, 99254, 99255, 99281, 99282, 99283, 99284, 99285, 99304, 99305, 99306, 99307, 99308, 99309, 99310, 99315, 99316, 99318, 99324, 99325, 99326, 99327, 99328, 99334, 99335, 99336, 99337, 99341, 99342, 99343, 99344, 99345, 99347, 99348, 99349, 99350, 99381-99397, 99495, 99496).◀

E/M 99202-99499

99497 Advance care planning including the explanation and discussion of advance directives such as standard forms (with completion of such forms, when performed), by the physician or other qualified health care professional; first 30 minutes, face-to-face with the patient, family member(s), and/or surrogate

➲ *CPT Changes: An Insider's View* 2015

➲ *CPT Assistant* Dec 14:11, Feb 16:7

+ 99498 each additional 30 minutes (List separately in addition to code for primary procedure)

➲ *CPT Changes: An Insider's View* 2015

➲ *CPT Assistant* Dec 14:11, Feb 16:7

(Use 99498 in conjunction with 99497)

(Do not report 99497 and 99498 on the same date of service as 99291, 99292, 99468, 99469, 99471, 99472, 99475, 99476, 99477, 99478, 99479, 99480, 99483)

General Behavioral Health Integration Care Management

►General behavioral health integration care management services (99484) are reported by the supervising physician or other qualified health care professional. The services are performed by clinical staff for a patient with a behavioral health (including substance use) condition that requires care management services (face-to-face or non-face-to-face) of 20 or more minutes in a calendar month. A treatment plan as well as the specified elements of the service description is required. The assessment and treatment plan is not required to be comprehensive and the office/practice is not required to have all the functions of chronic care management (99439, 99487, 99489, 99490). Code 99484 may be used in any outpatient setting, as long as the reporting professional has an ongoing relationship with the patient and clinical staff and as long as the clinical staff is available for face-to-face services with the patient.◄

The reporting professional must be able to perform the evaluation and management (E/M) services of an initiating visit. General behavioral integration care management (99484) and chronic care management services may be reported by the same professional in the same month, as long as distinct care management services are performed. Behavioral health integration care management (99484) and psychiatric collaborative care management (99492, 99493, 99494) may not be reported by the same professional in the same month. Behavioral health care integration clinical staff are not required to have qualifications that would permit them to separately report services (eg, psychotherapy), but, if qualified and they perform such services, they may report such services separately, as long as the time of the service is not used in reporting 99484.

 # 99484 Care management services for behavioral health conditions, at least 20 minutes of clinical staff time, directed by a physician or other qualified health care professional, per calendar month, with the following required elements:

- initial assessment or follow-up monitoring, including the use of applicable validated rating scales;
- behavioral health care planning in relation to behavioral/psychiatric health problems, including revision for patients who are not progressing or whose status changes;
- facilitating and coordinating treatment such as psychotherapy, pharmacotherapy, counseling and/or psychiatric consultation; and
- continuity of care with a designated member of the care team.

➲ *CPT Changes: An Insider's View* 2018

➲ *CPT Assistant* Feb 18:7, Mar 18:5, Jul 18:12, Feb 20:7

(Do not report 99484 in conjunction with 99492, 99493, 99494 in the same calendar month)

E/M 99202-99499

▶(E/M services, including care management services [99439, 99487, 99489, 99490, 99495, 99496], and psychiatric services [90785-90899] may be reported separately by the same physician or other qualified health care professional on the same day or during the same calendar month, but time and activities used to meet criteria for another reported service do not count toward meeting criteria for 99484)◀

Coding Tip

If the treating physician or other qualified health care professional personally performs behavioral health care manager activities and those activities are not used to meet the criteria for a separately reported code, his or her time may be counted toward the required behavioral health care manager time to meet the elements of 99484, 99492, 99493, 99494.

Clinical staff time spent coordinating care with the emergency department may be reported using 99484, but time spent while the patient is inpatient or admitted to observation status may not be reported using 99484.

Other Evaluation and Management Services

99499 **Unlisted evaluation and management** service

➲ *CPT Assistant* Apr 96:11, Mar 05:11, May 05:1, Jan 06:46, Sep 06:8, Jan 07:30, May 11:7, Apr 12:10, Jul 12:10, 11, Nov 12:13, Oct 14:9, Aug 19:8

SECTION 6

Appendixes A and B

2021

2020

This section consists of two appendixes and is intended to provide a useful guide to the evaluation and management (E/M) guideline revisions described thus far, as well as additional resources and other related materials to consult for additional information.

The objectives of this section are as follows:

- Use Appendix A for a detailed tabular review of changes in the E/M Sevices Guidelines for 2021, including additions, deletions, and revisions
- Use Appendix B for additional online resources and other related materials for the CPT 2021 E/M changes

APPENDIX A

Tabular Review of E/M Guideline Changes for 2021

In addition to the new sections for office or other outpatient E/M visits, it is important to remember that many of the existing guidelines are still in effect for other E/M categories; therefore, much of the existing guideline text remains, but has been relocated.

To assist users who wish to have a detailed review of the changes in the guidelines for 2021, a table of these changes (additions, revisions, relocations, and deletions for 2021), as they were constructed by the CPT Editorial Panel, is provided (see Table A2) together with a table that includes the symbols used in the table and what they mean (see Table A1).

TABLE A1 Annotation Symbols Used in the Tabular Review of E/M Guideline Changes for 2021

Annotation Symbol	Meaning
New	Indicates new text or heading. In addition, all new text appears underlined.
Revised	Indicates that some or all of the text has been revised. In addition, all revised text appears underlined.
Relocated	Indicates that the text has been relocated *to* a new area of the guidelines. The next column indicates the heading under which the text appeared in the pre-2021 guidelines (From), and the heading under which it has been placed in the 2021 guidelines (To).
▶ Relocated	Indicates the new location of the text that has been relocated *from* another area of the guidelines. The next column indicates the location of the text in the pre-2021 guidelines.
Deleted	Indicates that the text has been deleted from the guidelines for 2021. In addition, all deleted text appears with a ~~strikethrough~~.

TABLE A2 Tabular Review of E/M Guideline Changes for 2021

E/M Guideline Changes	Action	From/To (for Relocated Text)
Evaluation and Management (E/M) Services Guidelines		
In addition to the information presented in the Introduction, several other items unique to this section are defined or identified here.		
▶**E/M Guidelines Overview**◀	New	
▶The E/M guidelines have sections that are common to all E/M categories and sections that are category specific. Most of the categories and many of the subcategories of service have special guidelines or instructions unique to that category or subcategory. Where these are indicated, eg, "Inpatient Hospital Care," special instructions are presented before the listing of the specific E/M services codes. It is important to review the instructions for each category or subcategory. These guidelines are to be used by the reporting physician or other qualified health care professional to select the appropriate level of service. These guidelines do not establish documentation requirements or standards of care. The main purpose of documentation is to support care of the patient by current and future health care team(s).◀	New	
▶There are two sets of guidelines: one for office or other outpatient services and another for the remaining E/M services. There are sections that are common to both (ie, Guidelines in Common). These guidelines are presented as Guidelines Common to all E/M Services, Guidelines for E/M Services (Hospital Observation, Hospital Inpatient, Consultations, Emergency Department, Nursing Facility, Domiciliary, Rest Home, or Custodial Care, Home) and Guidelines for Office or Other Outpatient Services.◀	New	
▶The main differences between the two sets of guidelines is that the office or other outpatient services use medical decision making (MDM) ***or*** time as the basis for selecting a code level, whereas the other E/M codes use history, examination, ***and*** MDM and only use time when counseling and/or coordination of care dominates the service. The definitions of time are different for different categories of services.◀	New	

Appendix A

E/M Guideline Changes	Action	From/To (for Relocated Text)

▶Summary of Guideline Differences◀

▶Component(s) for Code Selection	Office or Other Outpatient Services	Other E/M Services (Hospital Observation, Hospital Inpatient, Consultations, Emergency Department, Nursing Facility, Domiciliary, Rest Home, or Custodial Care, Home)
History and Examination	• As medically appropriate. Not used in code selection	• Use key components (history, examination, MDM)
Medical Decision Making (MDM)	• May use MDM or total time on the date of the encounter	• Use key components (history, examination, MDM)
Time	• May use MDM or total time on the date of the encounter	• May use face-to-face or time at the bedside and on the patient's floor or unit when counseling and/or coordination of care dominates the service. *Time is **not** a descriptive component for the emergency department levels of E/M services.*
MDM Elements	• Number and complexity of problems addressed at the encounter • Amount and/or complexity of data to be reviewed and analyzed • Risk of complications and/or morbidity or mortality of patient management	• Number of diagnoses or management options • Amount and/or complexity of data to be reviewed • Risk of complications and/or morbidity or mortality◀

Action: New

Classification of Evaluation and Management (E/M) Services

▶The E/M section is divided into broad categories such as office visits, hospital visits, and consultations. Most of the categories are further divided into two or more subcategories of E/M services. For example, there are two subcategories of office visits (new patient and established patient) and there are two subcategories of hospital visits (initial and subsequent). The subcategories of E/M services are further classified into levels of E/M services that are identified by specific codes. ~~This classification is important because the nature of work varies by type of service, place of service, and the patient's status.~~◀

Action: Revised

Appendix A

E/M Guideline Changes	Action	From/To (for Relocated Text)
▶The basic format of the levels of E/M services is the same for most categories. First, a unique code number is listed. Second, the place and/or type of service is specified, eg, office consultation. Third, the content of the service is defined~~, eg, comprehensive history and comprehensive examination. (See "Levels of E/M Services," page 6, for details on the content of E/M services.)~~ Fourth~~, the nature of the presenting problem(s) usually associated with a given level is described. Fifth~~, ~~the~~ time ~~typically required to provide the service~~ is specified. (A detailed discussion of time is provided ~~on page 7~~following the Decision Tree for New vs Established Patients.)◀	Revised	
Definitions of Commonly Used Terms		
▶Certain key words and phrases are used throughout the E/M section. The following definitions are intended to reduce the potential for differing interpretations and to increase the consistency of reporting by physicians ~~in differing specialties. E/M services may also be reported by~~and other qualified health care professionals~~ who are authorized to perform such services within~~. The definitions in the E/M section are provided solely for the ~~scope~~basis of ~~their practice~~ code selection. ◀	Revised	
▶Some definitions are common to all categories of services and others are specific to one or more categories only.◀	New	

E/M Guideline Changes	Action	From/To (for Relocated Text)
~~**New and Established Patient**~~	Relocated	**From:** Definitions of Commonly Used Terms **To:** Guidelines Common to All E/M Services
~~Solely for the purposes of distinguishing between new and established patients, **professional services** are those face-to-face services rendered by physicians and other qualified health care professionals who may report evaluation and management services reported by a specific CPT code(s). A new patient is one who has not received any professional services from the physician/qualified health care professional or another physician/qualified health care professional of the **exact** same specialty **and subspecialty** who belongs to the same group practice, within the past three years.~~	Relocated	
~~An established patient is one who has received professional services from the physician/qualified health care professional or another physician/qualified health care professional of the **exact** same specialty **and subspecialty** who belongs to the same group practice, within the past three years. See Decision Tree.~~	Relocated	
~~In the instance where a physician/qualified health care professional is on call for or covering for another physician/qualified health care professional, the patient's encounter will be classified as it would have been by the physician/qualified health care professional who is not available. When advanced practice nurses and physician assistants are working with physicians they are considered as working in the exact same specialty and exact same subspecialties as the physician.~~	Relocated	
~~No distinction is made between new and established patients in the emergency department. E/M services in the emergency department category may be reported for any new or established patient who presents for treatment in the emergency department.~~	Relocated	
~~The Decision Tree on page 5 is provided to aid in determining whether to report the E/M service provided as a new or an established patient encounter.~~	Relocated Revised	
~~**Chief Complaint**~~	Relocated	**From:** Definitions of Commonly Used Terms **To:** Guidelines for Hospital Observation, Hospital Inpatient, Consultations, Emergency Department, Nursing Facility, Domiciliary, Rest Home, or Custodial Care, and Home E/M Services
~~A chief complaint is a concise statement describing the symptom, problem, condition, diagnosis, or other factor that is the reason for the encounter, usually stated in the patient's words.~~	Relocated	

E/M Guideline Changes	Action	From/To (for Relocated Text)
~~**Concurrent Care and Transfer of Care**~~	Relocated	From: Definitions of Commonly Used Terms To: Guidelines Common to All E/M Services
~~Concurrent care is the provision of similar services (eg, hospital visits) to the same patient by more than one physician or other qualified health care professional on the same day. When concurrent care is provided, no special reporting is required. Transfer of care is the process whereby a physician or other qualified health care professional who is providing management for some or all of a patient's problems relinquishes this responsibility to another physician or other qualified health care professional who explicitly agrees to accept this responsibility and who, from the initial encounter, is not providing consultative services. The physician or other qualified health care professional transferring care is then no longer providing care for these problems though he or she may continue providing care for other conditions when appropriate. Consultation codes should not be reported by the physician or other qualified health care professional who has agreed to accept transfer of care before an initial evaluation but are appropriate to report if the decision to accept transfer of care cannot be made until after the initial consultation evaluation, regardless of site of service.~~	Relocated	
~~**Counseling**~~	Relocated	From: Definitions of Commonly Used Terms To: Guidelines Common to All E/M Services
~~Counseling is a discussion with a patient and/or family concerning one or more of the following areas:~~ - ~~Diagnostic results, impressions, and/or recommended diagnostic studies~~ - ~~Prognosis~~ - ~~Risks and benefits of management (treatment) options~~ - ~~Instructions for management (treatment) and/or follow-up~~ - ~~Importance of compliance with chosen management (treatment) options~~ - ~~Risk factor reduction~~ - ~~Patient and family education~~	Relocated	
~~(For psychotherapy, see 90832-90834, 90836-90840)~~	Relocated	

E/M Guideline Changes	Action	From/To (for Relocated Text)
~~**Family History**~~	Relocated	**From:** Definitions of Commonly Used Terms **To:** Guidelines for Hospital Observation, Hospital Inpatient, Consultations, Emergency Department, Nursing Facility, Domiciliary, Rest Home, or Custodial Care, and Home E/M Services
~~A review of medical events in the patient's family that includes significant information about:~~ ▪ ~~The health status or cause of death of parents, siblings, and children~~ ▪ ~~Specific diseases related to problems identified in the Chief Complaint or History of the Present Illness, and/or System Review~~ ▪ ~~Diseases of family members that may be hereditary or place the patient at risk~~	Relocated	
~~**History of Present Illness**~~	Relocated	
~~A chronological description of the development of the patient's present illness from the first sign and/or symptom to the present. This includes a description of location, quality, severity, timing, context, modifying factors, and associated signs and symptoms significantly related to the presenting problem(s).~~	Relocated	
~~**Levels of E/M Services**~~	Relocated	**From:** Definitions of Commonly Used Terms **To:** Guidelines Common to All E/M Services
~~Within each category or subcategory of E/M service, there are three to five levels of E/M services available for reporting purposes. Levels of E/M services are **not** interchangeable among the different categories or subcategories of service. For example, the first level of E/M services in the subcategory of office visit, new patient, does not have the same definition as the first level of E/M services in the subcategory of office visit, established patient. Each level of E/M services may be used by all physicians or other qualified health care professionals.~~	Relocated	
~~The levels of E/M services include examinations, evaluations, treatments, conferences with or concerning patients, preventive pediatric and adult health supervision, and similar medical services, such as the determination of the need and/or location for appropriate care. Medical screening includes the history, examination, and medical decision making required to determine the need and/or location for appropriate care and treatment of the patient (eg, office and other outpatient setting, emergency department, nursing facility). The levels of E/M services encompass the wide variations in skill, effort, time, responsibility, and medical knowledge required for the prevention or diagnosis and treatment of illness or injury and the promotion of optimal health. Each level of E/M services may be used by all physicians or other qualified health care professionals.~~	All but last sentence Deleted last sentence Relocated	**From:** Definitions of Commonly Used Terms **To:** Guidelines Common to All E/M Services

E/M Guideline Changes	**Action**	**From/To (for Relocated Text)**
~~The descriptors for the levels of E/M services recognize seven components, six of which are used in defining the levels of E/M services. These components are:~~ ▪ ~~History~~ ▪ ~~Examination~~ ▪ ~~Medical decision making~~ ▪ ~~Counseling~~ ▪ ~~Coordination of care~~ ▪ ~~Nature of presenting problem~~ ▪ ~~Time~~	**Relocated**	**From:** Definitions of Commonly Used Terms **To:** Guidelines for Hospital Observation, Hospital Inpatient, Consultations, Emergency Department, Nursing Facility, Domiciliary, Rest Home, or Custodial Care, and Home E/M Services
~~The first three of these components (history, examination, and medical decision making) are considered the key components in selecting a level of E/M services. (See "Determine the Extent of History Obtained," page 9.)~~	**Relocated**	
~~The next three components (counseling, coordination of care, and the nature of the presenting problem) are considered contributory factors in the majority of encounters. Although the first two of these contributory factors are important E/M services, it is not required that these services be provided at every patient encounter.~~	**Relocated**	
~~Coordination of care with other physicians, other health care professionals, or agencies without a patient encounter on that day is reported using the case management codes.~~	**Relocated**	
~~The final component, time, is discussed in detail on page 7.~~	**Relocated**	

E/M Guideline Changes	Action	From/To (for Relocated Text)
~~Any specifically identifiable procedure (ie, identified with a specific CPT code) performed on or subsequent to the date of initial or subsequent E/M services should be reported separately.~~	Relocated	**From:** Definitions of Commonly Used Terms **To:** Guidelines Common to All E/M Services/ Services Reported Separately
~~The actual performance and/or interpretation of diagnostic tests/ studies ordered during a patient encounter are not included in the levels of E/M services. Physician performance of diagnostic tests/ studies for which specific CPT codes are available may be reported separately, in addition to the appropriate E/M code. The physician's interpretation of the results of diagnostic tests/studies (ie, professional component) with preparation of a separate distinctly identifiable signed written report may also be reported separately, using the appropriate CPT code with modifier 26 appended.~~	Relocated	
~~The physician or other health care professional may need to indicate that on the day a procedure or service identified by a CPT code was performed, the patient's condition required a significant separately identifiable E/M service above and beyond other services provided or beyond the usual preservice and postservice care associated with the procedure that was performed. The E/M service may be caused or prompted by the symptoms or condition for which the procedure and/or service was provided. This circumstance may be reported by adding modifier 25 to the appropriate level of E/M service. As such, different diagnoses are not required for reporting of the procedure and the E/M services on the same date.~~	Relocated	

E/M Guideline Changes	Action	From/To (for Relocated Text)
~~**Nature of Presenting Problem**~~	Relocated	
~~A presenting problem is a disease, condition, illness, injury, symptom, sign, finding, complaint, or other reason for encounter, with or without a diagnosis being established at the time of the encounter. The E/M codes recognize five types of presenting problems that are defined as follows:~~	Relocated	
~~***Minimal:*** A problem that may not require the presence of the physician or other qualified health care professional, but service is provided under the physician's or other qualified health care professional's supervision.~~	Relocated	**From:** Definitions of Commonly Used Terms **To:** Guidelines for Hospital Observation, Hospital Inpatient, Consultations, Emergency Department, Nursing Facility, Domiciliary, Rest Home, or Custodial Care, and Home E/M Services
~~***Self-limited or minor:*** A problem that runs a definite and prescribed course, is transient in nature, and is not likely to permanently alter health status OR has a good prognosis with management/compliance.~~	Revised Relocated	
~~***Low severity:*** A problem where the risk of morbidity without treatment is low; there is little to no risk of mortality without treatment; full recovery without functional impairment is expected.~~	Relocated	
~~***Moderate severity:*** A problem where the risk of morbidity without treatment is moderate; there is moderate risk of mortality without treatment; uncertain prognosis OR increased probability of prolonged functional impairment.~~	Relocated	
~~***High severity:*** A problem where the risk of morbidity without treatment is high to extreme; there is a moderate to high risk of mortality without treatment OR high probability of severe, prolonged functional impairment.~~	Relocated	
~~**Past History**~~	Relocated	**From:** Definitions of Commonly Used Terms
~~A review of the patient's past experiences with illnesses, injuries, and treatments that includes significant information about:~~ ▪ ~~Prior major illnesses and injuries~~ ▪ ~~Prior operations~~ ▪ ~~Prior hospitalizations~~ ▪ ~~Current medications~~ ▪ ~~Allergies (eg, drug, food)~~ ▪ ~~Age appropriate immunization status~~ ▪ ~~Age appropriate feeding/dietary status~~	Relocated	**To:** Guidelines for Hospital Observation, Hospital Inpatient, Consultations, Emergency Department, Nursing Facility, Domiciliary, Rest Home, or Custodial Care, and Home E/M Services

E/M Guideline Changes	Action	From/To (for Relocated Text)
~~**Social History**~~	Relocated	**From:** Definitions of Commonly Used Terms **To:** Guidelines for Hospital Observation, Hospital Inpatient, Consultations, Emergency Department, Nursing Facility, Domiciliary, Rest Home, or Custodial Care, and Home E/M Services
~~An age appropriate review of past and current activities that includes significant information about:~~ • ~~Marital status and/or living arrangements~~ • ~~Current employment~~ • ~~Occupational history~~ • ~~Military history~~ • ~~Use of drugs, alcohol, and tobacco~~ • ~~Level of education~~ • ~~Sexual history~~ • ~~Other relevant social factors~~	Relocated	
~~**System Review (Review of Systems)**~~	Relocated	**From:** Definitions of Commonly Used Terms **To:** Guidelines for Hospital Observation, Hospital Inpatient, Consultations, Emergency Department, Nursing Facility, Domiciliary, Rest Home, or Custodial Care, and Home E/M Services
~~An inventory of body systems obtained through a series of questions seeking to identify signs and/or symptoms that the patient may be experiencing or has experienced. For the purposes of the CPT codebook the following elements of a system review have been identified:~~ • ~~Constitutional symptoms (fever, weight loss, etc)~~ • ~~Eyes~~ • ~~Ears, nose, mouth, throat~~ • ~~Cardiovascular~~ • ~~Respiratory~~ • ~~Gastrointestinal~~ • ~~Genitourinary~~ • ~~Musculoskeletal~~ • ~~Integumentary (skin and/or breast)~~ • ~~Neurological~~ • ~~Psychiatric~~ • ~~Endocrine~~ • ~~Hematologic/lymphatic~~ • ~~Allergic/immunologic~~	Relocated	
~~The review of systems helps define the problem, clarify the differential diagnosis, identify needed testing, or serves as baseline data on other systems that might be affected by any possible management options.~~	Relocated	

E/M Guideline Changes	Action	From/To (for Relocated Text)
~~**Time**~~	Relocated	
~~The inclusion of time in the definitions of levels of E/M services has been implicit in prior editions of the CPT codebook. The inclusion of time as an explicit factor beginning in CPT 1992 is done to assist in selecting the most appropriate level of E/M services. It should be recognized that the specific times expressed in the visit code descriptors are averages and, therefore, represent a range of times that may be higher or lower depending on actual clinical circumstances.~~	Relocated	**From:** Definitions of Commonly Used Terms **To:** Guidelines Common to All E/M Services
~~Time is **not** a descriptive component for the emergency department levels of E/M services because emergency department services are typically provided on a variable intensity basis, often involving multiple encounters with several patients over an extended period of time. Therefore, it is often difficult to provide accurate estimates of the time spent face-to-face with the patient.~~	Relocated	
~~Studies to establish levels of E/M services employed surveys of practicing physicians to obtain data on the amount of time and work associated with typical E/M services. Since "work" is not easily quantifiable, the codes must rely on other objective, verifiable measures that correlate with physicians' estimates of their "work." It has been demonstrated that estimations of **intraservice** time (as explained on the next page), both within and across specialties, is a variable that is predictive of the "work" of E/M services. This same research has shown there is a strong relationship between intraservice time and total time for E/M services. Intraservice time, rather than total time, was chosen for inclusion with the codes because of its relative ease of measurement and because of its direct correlation with measurements of the total amount of time and work associated with typical E/M services.~~	Deleted	
~~Intraservice times are defined as face-to-face time for office and other outpatient visits and as unit/floor time for hospital and other inpatient visits. This distinction is necessary because most of the work of typical office visits takes place during the face-to-face time with the patient, while most of the work of typical hospital visits takes place during the time spent on the patient's floor or unit. When prolonged time occurs in either the office or the inpatient areas, the appropriate add-on code should be reported.~~	Deleted	
~~Face-to-face time (office and other outpatient visits and office consultations): For coding purposes, face-to-face time for these services is defined as only that time spent face-to-face with the patient and/or family. This includes the time spent performing such tasks as obtaining a history, examination, and counseling the patient.~~	Relocated	**From:** Definitions of Commonly Used Terms **To:** Guidelines Common to All E/M Services

E/M Guideline Changes	Action	From/To (for Relocated Text)
~~Time is also spent doing work before or after the face-to-face time with the patient, performing such tasks as reviewing records and tests, arranging for further services, and communicating further with other professionals and the patient through written reports and telephone contact.~~	Deleted	
~~This **non-face-to-face** time for office services—also called pre- and postencounter time—is not included in the time component described in the E/M codes. However, the pre- and post-non-face-to-face work associated with an encounter was included in calculating the total work of typical services in physician surveys.~~	Deleted	
~~Thus, the face-to-face time associated with the services described by any E/M code is a valid proxy for the total work done before, during, and after the visit.~~	Deleted	
~~***Unit/floor time (hospital observation services, inpatient hospital care, initial inpatient hospital consultations, nursing facility):*** For reporting purposes, intraservice time for these services is defined as unit/floor time, which includes the time present on the patient's hospital unit and at the bedside rendering services for that patient. This includes the time to establish and/or review the patient's chart, examine the patient, write notes, and communicate with other professionals and the patient's family.~~	Relocated	**From:** Definitions of Commonly Used Terms **To:** Guidelines Common to All E/M Services
~~In the hospital, pre- and post-time includes time spent off the patient's floor performing such tasks as reviewing pathology and radiology findings in another part of the hospital.~~	Deleted	
~~This pre- and postvisit time is not included in the time component described in these codes. However, the pre- and postwork performed during the time spent off the floor or unit was included in calculating the total work of typical services in physician surveys.~~	Deleted	
~~Thus, the unit/floor time associated with the services described by any code is a valid proxy for the total work done before, during, and after the visit.~~	Deleted	
▸**Guidelines Common to All E/M Services**◂	New	
▸**Levels of E/M Services**◂	New	
Within each category or subcategory of E/M service, there are three to five levels of E/M services available for reporting purposes. Levels of E/M services are **not** interchangeable among the different categories or subcategories of service. For example, the first level of E/M services in the subcategory of office visit, new patient, does not have the same definition as the first level of E/M services in the subcategory of office visit, established patient. Each level of E/M services may be used by all physicians or other qualified health care professionals.	Last sentence of paragraph Relocated	**Last sentence of 1st paragraph moved from:** Definitions of Commonly Used Terms

E/M Guideline Changes	Action	From/To (for Relocated Text)
New and Established Patient	Relocated	**From:** Definitions of Commonly Used Terms
Solely for the purposes of distinguishing between new and established patients, **professional services** are those face-to-face services rendered by physicians and other qualified health care professionals who may report evaluation and management services reported by a specific CPT code(s). A new patient is one who has not received any professional services from the physician/qualified health care professional or another physician/qualified health care professional of the **exact** same specialty **and subspecialty** who belongs to the same group practice, within the past three years.	Relocated	
An established patient is one who has received professional services from the physician/qualified health care professional or another physician/qualified health care professional of the **exact** same specialty **and subspecialty** who belongs to the same group practice, within the past three years. See Decision Tree for New vs Established Patients.	Relocated	
In the instance where a physician/qualified health care professional is on call for or covering for another physician/qualified health care professional, the patient's encounter will be classified as it would have been by the physician/qualified health care professional who is not available. When advanced practice nurses and physician assistants are working with physicians they are considered as working in the exact same specialty and exact same subspecialties as the physician.	Relocated	

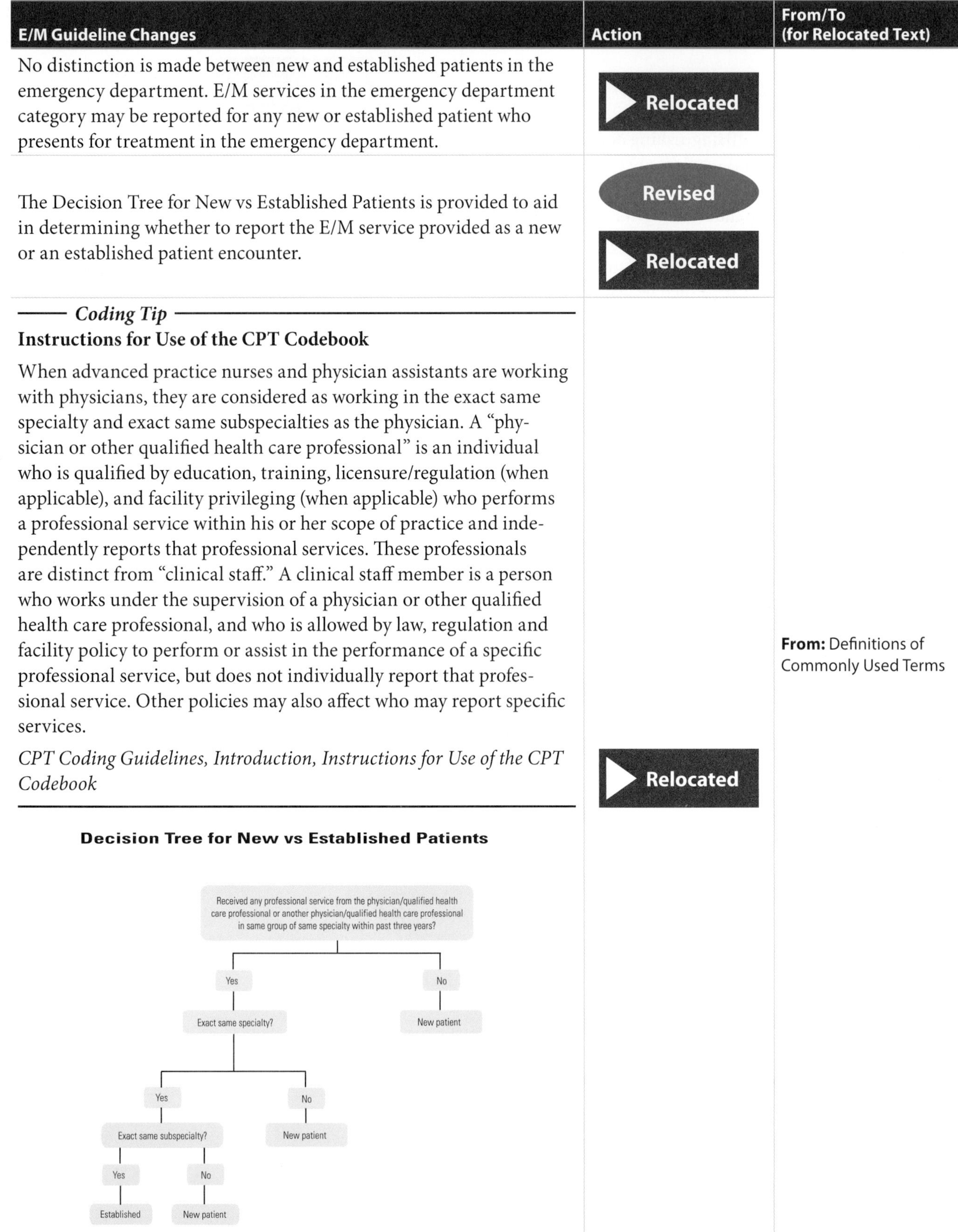

E/M Guideline Changes	Action	From/To (for Relocated Text)
No distinction is made between new and established patients in the emergency department. E/M services in the emergency department category may be reported for any new or established patient who presents for treatment in the emergency department.	Relocated	
The Decision Tree for New vs Established Patients is provided to aid in determining whether to report the E/M service provided as a new or an established patient encounter.	Revised Relocated	
Coding Tip **Instructions for Use of the CPT Codebook** When advanced practice nurses and physician assistants are working with physicians, they are considered as working in the exact same specialty and exact same subspecialties as the physician. A "physician or other qualified health care professional" is an individual who is qualified by education, training, licensure/regulation (when applicable), and facility privileging (when applicable) who performs a professional service within his or her scope of practice and independently reports that professional services. These professionals are distinct from "clinical staff." A clinical staff member is a person who works under the supervision of a physician or other qualified health care professional, and who is allowed by law, regulation and facility policy to perform or assist in the performance of a specific professional service, but does not individually report that professional service. Other policies may also affect who may report specific services. *CPT Coding Guidelines, Introduction, Instructions for Use of the CPT Codebook*		**From:** Definitions of Commonly Used Terms
Decision Tree for New vs Established Patients	Relocated	

E/M Guideline Changes	Action	From/To (for Relocated Text)
Time	Relocated	**From:** Definitions of Commonly Used Terms
▶The inclusion of time in the definitions of levels of E/M services has been implicit in prior editions of the CPT codebook. The inclusion of time as an explicit factor beginning in ~~*CPT 1992* is~~CPT 1992 was done to assist in selecting the most appropriate level of E/M services. ~~It should~~Beginning with CPT 2021, except for 99211, time alone may be ~~recognized that~~used to select the ~~specific times expressed in~~appropriate code level for the ~~visit code descriptors are averages and~~office or other outpatient E/M services codes (99202, 99203, 99204, 99205, 99212, 99213, ~~therefore~~99214, ~~represent a range~~99215). Different categories of ~~times that may be higher or lower depending on actual clinical circumstances~~services use time differently. It is important to review the instructions for each category.◀	Revised Relocated	**From:** Definitions of Commonly Used Terms
Time is **not** a descriptive component for the emergency department levels of E/M services because emergency department services are typically provided on a variable intensity basis, often involving multiple encounters with several patients over an extended period of time. Therefore, it is often difficult to provide accurate estimates of the time spent face-to-face with the patient.	Relocated	**From:** Definitions of Commonly Used Terms
▶Time may be used to select a code level in office or other outpatient services whether or not counseling and/or coordination of care dominates the service. Time may only be used for selecting the level of the ***other*** E/M services when counseling and/or coordination of care dominates the service.◀	New	
▶When time is used for reporting E/M services codes, the time defined in the service descriptors is used for selecting the appropriate level of services. The E/M services for which these guidelines apply require a face-to-face encounter with the physician or other qualified health care professional. For office or other outpatient services, if the physician's or other qualified health care professional's time is spent in the supervision of clinical staff who perform the face-to-face services of the encounter, use 99211.◀	New	
▶A shared or split visit is defined as a visit in which a physician and other qualified health care professional(s) jointly provide the face-to-face and non-face-to-face work related to the visit. When time is being used to select the appropriate level of services for which time-based reporting of shared or split visits is allowed, the time personally spent by the physician and other qualified health care professional(s) assessing and managing the patient on the date of the encounter is summed to define total time. Only distinct time should be summed for shared or split visits (ie, when two or more individuals jointly meet with or discuss the patient, only the time of one individual should be counted).◀	New	

E/M Guideline Changes	Action	From/To (for Relocated Text)
▶Intraservice times are defined as **face-to-face** time for office and other outpatient visits and as **unit/floor** time for hospital and other inpatient visits. This distinction is necessary because most of the work of typical office visits takes place during the face-to-faceWhen prolonged time with the patientoccurs, while most of the work of typical hospital visits takes place during theappropriate prolonged services code may be reported. The appropriate time spent on the patient's floor or unit. When prolonged time occursshould be documented in either the office or the inpatient areas,the medical record when it is used as the appropriate add-onbasis for code should be reportedselection.◀	Revised Relocated	**From:** Definitions of Commonly Used Terms
▶***Face-to-face time (office and other outpatient visitsoutpatient consultations [99241, 99242, 99243, 99244, 99245], domiciliary, rest home, or custodial services [99324, 99325, 99326, 99327, 99328, 99334, 99335, 99336, 99337], home services [99341, 99342, 99343, 99344, 99345, 99347, 99348, 99349, 99350], cognitive assessment and office consultationscare plan services [99483]):*** For coding purposes, face-to-face time for these services is defined as only that time spent face-to-face with the patient and/or family. This includes the time spent performing such tasks as obtaining a history, examination, and counseling the patient.◀	Revised Relocated	**From:** Definitions of Commonly Used Terms
▶***Unit/floor time (hospital observation services [99218, 99219, 99220, 99224, 99225, 99226, 99234, 99235, 99236], hospital inpatient hospital careservices [99221, 99222, 99223, 99231, 99232, initial99233], inpatient consultationshospital [99251, 99252, 99253, 99254, 99255], nursing facility services [99304, 99305, 99306, 99307, 99308, 99309, 99310, 99315, 99316, 99318]):*** For reportingcoding purposes, intraservice time for these services is defined as unit/floor time, which includes the time present on the patient's hospital unit and at the bedside rendering services for that patient. This includes the time to establish and/or review the patient's chart, examine the patient, write notes, and communicate with other professionals and the patient's family.◀	Revised Relocated	**From:** Definitions of Commonly Used Terms
▶***Total time on the date of the encounter (office or other outpatient services [99202, 99203, 99204, 99205, 99212, 99213, 99214, 99215]):*** For coding purposes, time for these services is the total time on the date of the encounter. It includes both the face-to-face and non-face-to-face time personally spent by the physician and/or other qualified health care professional(s) on the day of the encounter (includes time in activities that require the physician or other qualified health care professional and does not include time in activities normally performed by clinical staff).◀	New	

Appendix A

E/M Guideline Changes	Action	From/To (for Relocated Text)
▶Physician/other qualified health care professional time includes the following activities, when performed: ▪ preparing to see the patient (eg, review of tests) ▪ obtaining and/or reviewing separately obtained history ▪ performing a medically appropriate examination and/or evaluation ▪ counseling and educating the patient/family/caregiver ▪ ordering medications, tests, or procedures ▪ referring and communicating with other health care professionals (when not separately reported) ▪ documenting clinical information in the electronic or other health record ▪ independently interpreting results (not separately reported) and communicating results to the patient/family/caregiver ▪ care coordination (not separately reported)◀	New	
Concurrent Care and Transfer of Care	Relocated	From: Definitions of Commonly Used Terms
Concurrent care is the provision of similar services (eg, hospital visits) to the same patient by more than one physician or other qualified health care professional on the same day. When concurrent care is provided, no special reporting is required. Transfer of care is the process whereby a physician or other qualified health care professional who is providing management for some or all of a patient's problems relinquishes this responsibility to another physician or other qualified health care professional who explicitly agrees to accept this responsibility and who, from the initial encounter, is not providing consultative services. The physician or other qualified health care professional transferring care is then no longer providing care for these problems though he or she may continue providing care for other conditions when appropriate. Consultation codes should not be reported by the physician or other qualified health care professional who has agreed to accept transfer of care before an initial evaluation but are appropriate to report if the decision to accept transfer of care cannot be made until after the initial consultation evaluation, regardless of site of service.	Relocated	

E/M Guideline Changes	Action	From/To (for Relocated Text)
Counseling	Relocated	From: Definitions of Commonly Used Terms
Counseling is a discussion with a patient and/or family concerning one or more of the following areas: ▪ Diagnostic results, impressions, and/or recommended diagnostic studies ▪ Prognosis ▪ Risks and benefits of management (treatment) options ▪ Instructions for management (treatment) and/or follow-up ▪ Importance of compliance with chosen management (treatment) options ▪ Risk factor reduction ▪ Patient and family education	Relocated	
(For psychotherapy, see 90832-90834, 90836-90840)	Relocated	
▶**Services Reported Separately**◀	New	

E/M Guideline Changes	Action	From/To (for Relocated Text)
▶Any specifically identifiable procedure or service (ie, identified with a specific CPT code) performed on ~~or subsequent to~~ the date of ~~initial or subsequent~~ E/M services ~~should~~may be reported separately.◀	Revised Relocated	
▶The actual performance and/or interpretation of diagnostic tests/studies ~~ordered~~ during a patient encounter are not included in determining the levels of E/M services when reported separately. Physician performance of diagnostic tests/studies for which specific CPT codes are available may be reported separately, in addition to the appropriate E/M code. The physician's interpretation of the results of diagnostic tests/studies (ie, professional component) with preparation of a separate distinctly identifiable signed written report may also be reported separately, using the appropriate CPT code and, if required, with modifier 26 appended. If a test/study is independently interpreted in order to manage the patient as part of the E/M service, but is not separately reported, it is part of MDM.◀	Revised Relocated	**From:** Definitions of Commonly Used Terms/Levels of E/M Services
▶The physician or other qualified health care professional may need to indicate that on the day a procedure or service identified by a CPT code was performed, the patient's condition required a significant separately identifiable E/M service ~~above and beyond other services provided or beyond the usual preservice and postservice care associated with the procedure that was performed~~. The E/M service may be caused or prompted by the symptoms or condition for which the procedure and/or service was provided. This circumstance may be reported by adding modifier 25 to the appropriate level of E/M service. As such, different diagnoses are not required for reporting of the procedure and the E/M services on the same date.◀	Revised Relocated	
▶Guidelines for Hospital Observation, Hospital Inpatient, Consultations, Emergency Department, Nursing Facility, Domiciliary, Rest Home, or Custodial Care, and Home E/M Services◀	New	

E/M Guideline Changes	Action	From/To (for Relocated Text)
Levels of E/M Services	Relocated	**From:** Definitions of Commonly Used Terms/ Levels of E/M Services
The descriptors for the levels of E/M services recognize seven components, six of which are used in defining the levels of E/M services. These components are: ▪ History ▪ Examination ▪ Medical decision making ▪ Counseling ▪ Coordination of care ▪ Nature of presenting problem ▪ Time	Relocated	
The first three of these components (history, examination, and medical decision making) are considered the **key** components in selecting a level of E/M services. (See "Determine the Extent of History Obtained~~;~~." ~~page 9~~.)	Relocated	
The next three components (counseling, coordination of care, and the nature of the presenting problem) are considered **contributory** factors in the majority of encounters. Although the first two of these contributory factors are important E/M services, it is not required that these services be provided at every patient encounter.	Relocated	
Coordination of care with other physicians, other health care professionals, or agencies without a patient encounter on that day is reported using the case management codes.	Relocated	**From:** Definitions of Commonly Used Terms/ Levels of E/M Services
▶The final component, time, is discussed in detail ~~on page 7~~following the Decision Tree for New vs Established Patients.◀	Revised Relocated	
Chief Complaint	Relocated	**From:** Definitions of Commonly Used Terms
A chief complaint is a concise statement describing the symptom, problem, condition, diagnosis, or other factor that is the reason for the encounter, usually stated in the patient's words.	Relocated	
History of Present Illness	Relocated	**From:** Definitions of Commonly Used Terms
A chronological description of the development of the patient's present illness from the first sign and/or symptom to the present. This includes a description of location, quality, severity, timing, context, modifying factors, and associated signs and symptoms significantly related to the presenting problem(s).	Relocated	

E/M Guideline Changes	Action	From/To (for Relocated Text)
Nature of Presenting Problem	Relocated	
A presenting problem is a disease, condition, illness, injury, symptom, sign, finding, complaint, or other reason for encounter, with or without a diagnosis being established at the time of the encounter. The E/M codes recognize five types of presenting problems that are defined as follows:	Relocated	**From:** Definitions of Commonly Used Terms
Minimal: A problem that may not require the presence of the physician or other qualified health care professional, but service is provided under the physician's or other qualified health care professional's supervision.	Relocated	
▶***Self-limited or minor:*** A problem that runs a definite and prescribed course, is transient in nature, and is not likely to permanently alter health status ~~OR has a good prognosis with management/compliance.~~◀	Revised Relocated	
Low severity: A problem where the risk of morbidity without treatment is low; there is little to no risk of mortality without treatment; full recovery without functional impairment is expected.	Relocated	**From:** Definitions of Commonly Used Terms
Moderate severity: A problem where the risk of morbidity without treatment is moderate; there is moderate risk of mortality without treatment; uncertain prognosis OR increased probability of prolonged functional impairment.	Relocated	
High severity: A problem where the risk of morbidity without treatment is high to extreme; there is a moderate to high risk of mortality without treatment OR high probability of severe, prolonged functional impairment.	Relocated	
Past History	Relocated	
A review of the patient's past experiences with illnesses, injuries, and treatments that includes significant information about: ▪ Prior major illnesses and injuries ▪ Prior operations ▪ Prior hospitalizations ▪ Current medications ▪ Allergies (eg, drug, food) ▪ Age appropriate immunization status ▪ Age appropriate feeding/dietary status	Relocated	**From:** Definitions of Commonly Used Terms

E/M Guideline Changes	Action	From/To (for Relocated Text)
Family History	Relocated	From: Definitions of Commonly Used Terms
A review of medical events in the patient's family that includes significant information about: ▪ The health status or cause of death of parents, siblings, and children ▪ Specific diseases related to problems identified in the Chief Complaint or History of the Present Illness, and/or System Review ▪ Diseases of family members that may be hereditary or place the patient at risk	Relocated	
Social History	Relocated	From: Definitions of Commonly Used Terms
An age appropriate review of past and current activities that includes significant information about: ▪ Marital status and/or living arrangements ▪ Current employment ▪ Occupational history ▪ Military history ▪ Use of drugs, alcohol, and tobacco ▪ Level of education ▪ Sexual history ▪ Other relevant social factors	Relocated	

E/M Guideline Changes	Action	From/To (for Relocated Text)
System Review (Review of Systems)	Relocated	
An inventory of body systems obtained through a series of questions seeking to identify signs and/or symptoms that the patient may be experiencing or has experienced. For the purposes of the CPT codebook the following elements of a system review have been identified: ▪ Constitutional symptoms (fever, weight loss, etc) ▪ Eyes ▪ Ears, nose, mouth, throat ▪ Cardiovascular ▪ Respiratory ▪ Gastrointestinal ▪ Genitourinary ▪ Musculoskeletal ▪ Integumentary (skin and/or breast) ▪ Neurological ▪ Psychiatric ▪ Endocrine ▪ Hematologic/lymphatic ▪ Allergic/immunologic	Relocated	**From:** Definitions of Commonly Used Terms
The review of systems helps define the problem, clarify the differential diagnosis, identify needed testing, or serves as baseline data on other systems that might be affected by any possible management options.	Relocated	

E/M Guideline Changes	Action	From/To (for Relocated Text)
~~Unlisted Service~~	Relocated	
~~An E/M service may be provided that is not listed in this section of the CPT codebook. When reporting such a service, the appropriate unlisted code may be used to indicate the service, identifying it by "Special Report," as discussed in the following paragraph. The "Unlisted Services" and accompanying codes for the E/M section are as follows:~~ ~~**99429 Unlisted preventive** medicine service~~ ~~**99499 Unlisted evaluation and management** service~~	Relocated	
~~Special Report~~	Relocated	
~~An unlisted service or one that is unusual, variable, or new may require a special report demonstrating the medical appropriateness of the service. Pertinent information should include an adequate definition or description of the nature, extent, and need for the procedure and the time, effort, and equipment necessary to provide the service. Additional items that may be included are complexity of symptoms, final diagnosis, pertinent physical findings, diagnostic and therapeutic procedures, concurrent problems, and follow-up care.~~	Relocated	**From:** Middle of the Guidelines Section **To:** End of the Guidelines Section
~~Clinical Examples~~	Relocated	
~~Clinical examples of the codes for E/M services are provided to assist in understanding the meaning of the descriptors and selecting the correct code. The clinical examples are listed in Appendix C. Each example was developed by the specialties shown.~~	Relocated	
~~The same problem, when seen by different specialties, may involve different amounts of work. Therefore, the appropriate level of encounter should be reported using the descriptors rather than the examples.~~	Relocated	
~~The same problem, when seen by different specialties, may involve different amounts of work. Therefore, the appropriate level of encounter should be reported using the descriptors rather than the examples.~~	Relocated	
▸Instructions for Selecting a Level of E/M Service for Hospital Observation, Hospital Inpatient, Consultations, Emergency Department, Nursing Facility, Domiciliary, Rest Home, or Custodial Care, and Home E/M Services◂	Revised	

E/M Guideline Changes	Action	From/To (for Relocated Text)
~~Review the Reporting Instructions for the Selected Category or Subcategory~~	Deleted	
~~Most of the categories and many of the subcategories of service have special guidelines or instructions unique to that category or subcategory. Where these are indicated, eg, "Inpatient Hospital Care," special instructions will be presented preceding the levels of E/M services.~~	Deleted	
Review the Level of E/M Service Descriptors and Examples in the Selected Category or Subcategory		
The descriptors for the levels of E/M services recognize seven components, six of which are used in defining the levels of E/M services. These components are: ▪ History ▪ Examination ▪ Medical decision making ▪ Counseling ▪ Coordination of care ▪ Nature of presenting problem ▪ Time		
►The first three of these components (ie, history, examination, and medical decision making) should be considered the **key** components in selecting the level of E/M services. An exception to this rule is in the case of visits that consist predominantly of counseling or coordination of care ~~(see numbered paragraph 3, page 10)~~.◄	Revised	
The nature of the presenting problem and time are provided in some levels to assist the physician in determining the appropriate level of E/M service.	No Change from Previous Position	
Determine the Extent of History Obtained	No Change from Previous Position	
The extent of the history is dependent upon clinical judgment and on the nature of the presenting problem(s). The levels of E/M services recognize four types of history that are defined as follows:	No Change from Previous Position	
Problem focused: Chief complaint; brief history of present illness or problem.	No Change from Previous Position	
Expanded problem focused: Chief complaint; brief history of present illness; problem pertinent system review.	No Change from Previous Position	
Detailed: Chief complaint; extended history of present illness; problem pertinent system review extended to include a review of a limited number of additional systems; **pertinent** past, family, and/or social history **directly related to the patient's problems.**	No Change from Previous Position	

E/M Guideline Changes	Action	From/To (for Relocated Text)
Comprehensive: Chief complaint; extended history of present illness; review of systems that is directly related to the problem(s) identified in the history of the present illness plus a review of all additional body systems; **complete** past, family, and social history.	**No Change from Previous Position**	
The comprehensive history obtained as part of the preventive medicine E/M service is not problem-oriented and does not involve a chief complaint or present illness. It does, however, include a comprehensive system review and comprehensive or interval past, family, and social history as well as a comprehensive assessment/history of pertinent risk factors.	**No Change from Previous Position**	
Determine the Extent of Examination Performed	**No Change from Previous Position**	
The extent of the examination performed is dependent on clinical judgment and on the nature of the presenting problem(s). The levels of E/M services recognize four types of examination that are defined as follows:	**No Change from Previous Position**	
Problem focused: A limited examination of the affected body area or organ system.	**No Change from Previous Position**	
Expanded problem focused: A limited examination of the affected body area or organ system and other symptomatic or related organ system(s).	**No Change from Previous Position**	
Detailed: An extended examination of the affected body area(s) and other symptomatic or related organ system(s).	**No Change from Previous Position**	
Comprehensive: A general multisystem examination or a complete examination of a single organ system. **Note:** The comprehensive examination performed as part of the preventive medicine E/M service is multisystem, but its extent is based on age and risk factors identified.	**No Change from Previous Position**	
For the purposes of these CPT definitions, the following body areas are recognized: ▪ Head, including the face ▪ Neck ▪ Chest, including breasts and axilla ▪ Abdomen ▪ Genitalia, groin, buttocks ▪ Back ▪ Each extremity	**No Change from Previous Position**	

E/M Guideline Changes	Action	From/To (for Relocated Text)
For the purposes of these CPT definitions, the following organ systems are recognized: ▪ Eyes ▪ Ears, nose, mouth, and throat ▪ Cardiovascular ▪ Respiratory ▪ Gastrointestinal ▪ Genitourinary ▪ Musculoskeletal ▪ Skin ▪ Neurologic ▪ Psychiatric ▪ Hematologic/lymphatic/immunologic	**No Change from Previous Position**	
Determine the Complexity of Medical Decision Making	**No Change from Previous Position**	
Medical decision making refers to the complexity of establishing a diagnosis and/or selecting a management option as measured by: ▪ The number of possible diagnoses and/or the number of management options that must be considered ▪ The amount and/or complexity of medical records, diagnostic tests, and/or other information that must be obtained, reviewed, and analyzed ▪ The risk of significant complications, morbidity, and/or mortality, as well as comorbidities, associated with the patient's presenting problem(s), the diagnostic procedure(s), and/or the possible management options	**No Change from Previous Position**	
Four types of medical decision making are recognized: straightforward, low complexity, moderate complexity, and high complexity. To qualify for a given type of decision making, two of the three elements in Table 1 must be met or exceeded.	**No Change from Previous Position**	
Comorbidities/underlying diseases, in and of themselves, are not considered in selecting a level of E/M services unless their presence significantly increases the complexity of the medical decision making.	**No Change from Previous Position**	
Select the Appropriate Level of E/M Services Based on the Following		

E/M Guideline Changes	Action	From/To (for Relocated Text)
▶1. For the following categories/subcategories, **all of the key components,** ie, history, examination, and medical decision making, must meet or exceed the stated requirements to qualify for a particular level of E/M service: ~~office, new patient~~initial observation care; initial hospital care; observation ~~services; initial~~or inpatient hospital care (including admission and discharge services); office or other outpatient consultations; ~~initial~~ inpatient consultations; emergency department services; initial nursing facility care; other nursing facility services; domiciliary care, new patient; and home services, new patient.◀	Revised	
▶2. For the following categories/subcategories, **two of the three key components** (ie, history, examination, and medical decision making) must meet or exceed the stated requirements to qualify for a particular level of E/M services: ~~office, established patient~~subsequent observation care; subsequent hospital care; subsequent nursing facility care; domiciliary care, established patient; and home services, established patient.◀	Revised	
3. When counseling and/or coordination of care dominates (more than 50%) the encounter with the patient and/or family (face-to-face time in the office or other outpatient setting or floor/unit time in the hospital or nursing facility), then **time** shall be considered the key or controlling factor to qualify for a particular level of E/M services. This includes time spent with parties who have assumed responsibility for the care of the patient or decision making whether or not they are family members (eg, foster parents, person acting in loco parentis, legal guardian). The extent of counseling and/or coordination of care must be documented in the medical record.	No Change from Previous Position	

Table 1
Complexity of Medical Decision Making

Number of Diagnoses or Management Options	Amount and/or Complexity of Data to be Reviewed	Risk of Complications and/or Morbidity or Mortality	Type of Decision Making
minimal	minimal or none	minimal	**straightforward**
limited	limited	low	**low complexity**
multiple	moderate	moderate	**moderate complexity**
extensive	extensive	high	**high complexity**

Action: No Change from Previous Position

▸Guidelines for Office or Other Outpatient E/M Services◂

Action: New

▸History and/or Examination◂

Action: New

E/M Guideline Changes	Action	From/To (for Relocated Text)
▶Office or other outpatient services include a medically appropriate history and/or physical examination, when performed. The nature and extent of the history and/or physical examination are determined by the treating physician or other qualified health care professional reporting the service. The care team may collect information and the patient or caregiver may supply information directly (eg, by electronic health record [EHR] portal or questionnaire) that is reviewed by the reporting physician or other qualified health care professional. The extent of history and physical examination is not an element in selection of office or other outpatient codes.◀	New	
▶**Number and Complexity of Problems Addressed at the Encounter**◀	New	
▶One element used in selecting the level of office or other outpatient services is the number and complexity of the problems that are addressed at an encounter. Multiple new or established conditions may be addressed at the same time and may affect MDM. Symptoms may cluster around a specific diagnosis and each symptom is not necessarily a unique condition. Comorbidities/underlying diseases, in and of themselves, are not considered in selecting a level of E/M services **unless** they are addressed, and their presence increases the amount and/or complexity of data to be reviewed and analyzed or the risk of complications and/or morbidity or mortality of patient management. The final diagnosis for a condition does not, in and of itself, determine the complexity or risk, as extensive evaluation may be required to reach the conclusion that the signs or symptoms do not represent a highly morbid condition. Multiple problems of a lower severity may, in the aggregate, create higher risk due to interaction.◀	New	
▶Definitions for the elements of MDM (see Table 2, Levels of Medical Decision Making) for office or other outpatient services are:◀	New	
▶***Problem:*** A problem is a disease, condition, illness, injury, symptom, sign, finding, complaint, or other matter addressed at the encounter, with or without a diagnosis being established at the time of the encounter.◀	New	

E/M Guideline Changes	Action	From/To (for Relocated Text)
▶***Problem addressed:*** A problem is addressed or managed when it is evaluated or treated at the encounter by the physician or other qualified health care professional reporting the service. This includes consideration of further testing or treatment that may not be elected by virtue of risk/benefit analysis or patient/parent/guardian/surrogate choice. Notation in the patient's medical record that another professional is managing the problem without additional assessment or care coordination documented does not qualify as being addressed or managed by the physician or other qualified health care professional reporting the service. Referral without evaluation (by history, examination, or diagnostic study[ies]) or consideration of treatment does not qualify as being addressed or managed by the physician or other qualified health care professional reporting the service.◀	New	
▶***Minimal problem:*** A problem that may not require the presence of the physician or other qualified health care professional, but the service is provided under the physician's or other qualified health care professional's supervision (see 99211).◀	New	
▶***Self-limited or minor problem:*** A problem that runs a definite and prescribed course, is transient in nature, and is not likely to permanently alter health status.◀	New	
▶***Stable, chronic illness:*** A problem with an expected duration of at least one year or until the death of the patient. For the purpose of defining chronicity, conditions are treated as chronic whether or not stage or severity changes (eg, uncontrolled diabetes and controlled diabetes are a single chronic condition). "Stable" for the purposes of categorizing MDM is defined by the specific treatment goals for an individual patient. A patient who is not at his or her treatment goal is not stable, even if the condition has not changed and there is no short-term threat to life or function. For example, in a patient with persistently poorly controlled blood pressure for whom better control is a goal is not stable, even if the pressures are not changing and the patient is asymptomatic, the risk of morbidity **without** treatment is significant. Examples may include well-controlled hypertension, non-insulin-dependent diabetes, cataract, or benign prostatic hyperplasia.◀	New	
▶***Acute, uncomplicated illness or injury:*** A recent or new short-term problem with low risk of morbidity for which treatment is considered. There is little to no risk of mortality with treatment, and full recovery without functional impairment is expected. A problem that is normally self-limited or minor but is not resolving consistent with a definite and prescribed course is an acute, uncomplicated illness. Examples may include cystitis, allergic rhinitis, or a simple sprain.◀	New	

E/M Guideline Changes	Action	From/To (for Relocated Text)
▶***Chronic illness with exacerbation, progression, or side effects of treatment:*** A chronic illness that is acutely worsening, poorly controlled, or progressing with an intent to control progression and requiring additional supportive care or requiring attention to treatment for side effects but that does not require consideration of hospital level of care.◀	New	
▶***Undiagnosed new problem with uncertain prognosis:*** A problem in the differential diagnosis that represents a condition likely to result in a high risk of morbidity without treatment. An example may be a lump in the breast.◀	New	
▶***Acute illness with systemic symptoms:*** An illness that causes systemic symptoms and has a high risk of morbidity without treatment. For systemic general symptoms, such as fever, body aches, or fatigue in a minor illness that may be treated to alleviate symptoms, shorten the course of illness, or to prevent complications, see the definitions for ***self-limited or minor problem*** or ***acute, uncomplicated illness or injury.*** Systemic symptoms may not be general but may be single system. Examples may include pyelonephritis, pneumonitis, or colitis.◀	New	
▶***Acute, complicated injury:*** An injury which requires treatment that includes evaluation of body systems that are not directly part of the injured organ, the injury is extensive, or the treatment options are multiple and/or associated with risk of morbidity. An example may be a head injury with brief loss of consciousness.◀	New	
▶***Chronic illness with severe exacerbation, progression, or side effects of treatment:*** The severe exacerbation or progression of a chronic illness or severe side effects of treatment that have significant risk of morbidity and may require hospital level of care.◀	New	
▶***Acute or chronic illness or injury that poses a threat to life or bodily function:*** An acute illness with systemic symptoms, an acute complicated injury, or a chronic illness or injury with exacerbation and/or progression or side effects of treatment, that poses a threat to life or bodily function in the near term without treatment. Examples may include acute myocardial infarction, pulmonary embolus, severe respiratory distress, progressive severe rheumatoid arthritis, psychiatric illness with potential threat to self or others, peritonitis, acute renal failure, or an abrupt change in neurologic status.◀	New	
▶***Test:*** Tests are imaging, laboratory, psychometric, or physiologic data. A clinical laboratory panel (eg, basic metabolic panel [80047]) is a single test. The differentiation between single or multiple unique tests is defined in accordance with the CPT code set.◀	New	
▶***External:*** External records, communications and/or test results are from an external physician, other qualified health care professional, facility, or health care organization.◀	New	

E/M Guideline Changes	Action	From/To (for Relocated Text)
▶***External physician or other qualified health care professional:*** An external physician or other qualified health care professional who is not in the same group practice or is of a different specialty or subspecialty. This includes licensed professionals who are practicing independently. The individual may also be a facility or organizational provider such as from a hospital, nursing facility, or home health care agency.◀	New	
▶***Independent historian(s):*** An individual (eg, parent, guardian, surrogate, spouse, witness) who provides a history in addition to a history provided by the patient who is unable to provide a complete or reliable history (eg, due to developmental stage, dementia, or psychosis) or because a confirmatory history is judged to be necessary. In the case where there may be conflict or poor communication between multiple historians and more than one historian is needed, the independent historian requirement is met.◀	New	
▶***Independent interpretation:*** The interpretation of a test for which there is a CPT code and an interpretation or report is customary. This does not apply when the physician or other qualified health care professional is reporting the service or has previously reported the service for the patient. A form of interpretation should be documented but need not conform to the usual standards of a complete report for the test.◀	New	
▶***Appropriate source:*** For the purpose of the **discussion of management** data element (see Table 2, Levels of Medical Decision Making), an appropriate source includes professionals who are not health care professionals but may be involved in the management of the patient (eg, lawyer, parole officer, case manager, teacher). It does not include discussion with family or informal caregivers.◀	New	
▶***Risk:*** The probability and/or consequences of an event. The assessment of the level of risk is affected by the nature of the event under consideration. For example, a low probability of death may be high risk, whereas a high chance of a minor, self-limited adverse effect of treatment may be low risk. Definitions of risk are based upon the usual behavior and thought processes of a physician or other qualified health care professional in the same specialty. Trained clinicians apply common language usage meanings to terms such as *high, medium, low,* or *minimal* risk and do not require quantification for these definitions (though quantification may be provided when evidence-based medicine has established probabilities). For the purposes of MDM, level of risk is based upon consequences of the problem(s) addressed at the encounter when appropriately treated. Risk also includes MDM related to the need to initiate or forego further testing, treatment, and/or hospitalization.◀	New	

E/M Guideline Changes	Action	From/To (for Relocated Text)
▶***Morbidity:*** A state of illness or functional impairment that is expected to be of substantial duration during which function is limited, quality of life is impaired, or there is organ damage that may not be transient despite treatment.◀	New	
▶***Social determinants of health:*** Economic and social conditions that influence the health of people and communities. Examples may include food or housing insecurity.◀	New	
▶***Drug therapy requiring intensive monitoring for toxicity:*** A drug that requires intensive monitoring is a therapeutic agent that has the potential to cause serious morbidity or death. The monitoring is performed for assessment of these adverse effects and not primarily for assessment of therapeutic efficacy. The monitoring should be that which is generally accepted practice for the agent but may be patient-specific in some cases. Intensive monitoring may be long-term or short-term. Long-term intensive monitoring is not performed less than quarterly. The monitoring may be performed with a laboratory test, a physiologic test, or imaging. Monitoring by history or examination does not qualify. The monitoring affects the level of MDM in an encounter in which it is considered in the management of the patient. Examples may include monitoring for cytopenia in the use of an antineoplastic agent between dose cycles or the short-term intensive monitoring of electrolytes and renal function in a patient who is undergoing diuresis. Examples of monitoring that do not qualify include monitoring glucose levels during insulin therapy, as the primary reason is the therapeutic effect (even if hypoglycemia is a concern); or annual electrolytes and renal function for a patient on a diuretic, as the frequency does not meet the threshold.◀	New	
▶**Instructions for Selecting a Level of Office or Other Outpatient E/M Services**◀	New	
▶Select the appropriate level of E/M services based on the following:◀	New	
▶1. The level of the MDM as defined for each service, **or**◀	New	
▶2. The total time for E/M services performed on the date of the encounter.◀	New	
▶**Medical Decision Making**◀	New	

Appendix A

<table>
<tr><th>E/M Guideline Changes</th><th>Action</th><th>From/To (for Relocated Text)</th></tr>
<tr><td>▶MDM includes establishing diagnoses, assessing the status of a condition, and/or selecting a management option. MDM in the office or other outpatient services codes is defined by three elements:
▪ The number and complexity of problem(s) that are addressed during the encounter.
▪ The amount and/or complexity of data to be reviewed and analyzed. These data include medical records, tests, and/or other information that must be obtained, ordered, reviewed, and analyzed for the encounter. This includes information obtained from multiple sources or interprofessional communications that are not reported separately and interpretation of tests that are not reported separately. Ordering a test is included in the category of test result(s) and the review of the test result is part of the encounter and not a subsequent encounter. Data are divided into three categories:
• Tests, documents, orders, or independent historian(s). (Each unique test, order, or document is counted to meet a threshold number.)
• Independent interpretation of tests.
• Discussion of management or test interpretation with external physician or other qualified health care professional or appropriate source.
▪ The risk of complications and/or morbidity or mortality of patient management decisions made at the visit, associated with the patient's problem(s), the diagnostic procedure(s), treatment(s). This includes the possible management options selected and those considered but not selected, after shared MDM with the patient and/or family. For example, a decision about hospitalization includes consideration of alternative levels of care. Examples may include a psychiatric patient with a sufficient degree of support in the outpatient setting or the decision to not hospitalize a patient with advanced dementia with an acute condition that would generally warrant inpatient care, but for whom the goal is palliative treatment.◀</td><td>New</td><td></td></tr>
<tr><td>▶Four types of MDM are recognized: straightforward, low, moderate, and high. The concept of the level of MDM does not apply to 99211.◀</td><td>New</td><td></td></tr>
<tr><td>▶Shared MDM involves eliciting patient and/or family preferences, patient and/or family education, and explaining risks and benefits of management options.◀</td><td>New</td><td></td></tr>
<tr><td>▶MDM may be impacted by role and management responsibility.◀</td><td>New</td><td></td></tr>
</table>

E/M Guideline Changes	Action	From/To (for Relocated Text)
▶When the physician or other qualified health care professional is reporting a separate CPT code that includes interpretation and/or report, the interpretation and/or report should not count toward the MDM when selecting a level of office or other outpatient services. When the physician or other qualified health care professional is reporting a separate service for discussion of management with a physician or another qualified health care professional, the discussion is not counted toward the MDM when selecting a level of office or other outpatient services.◀	New	
▶The Levels of Medical Decision Making (MDM) table (Table 2) is a guide to assist in selecting the level of MDM for reporting an office or other outpatient E/M services code. The table includes the four levels of MDM (ie, straightforward, low, moderate, high) and the three elements of MDM (ie, number and complexity of problems addressed at the encounter, amount and/or complexity of data reviewed and analyzed, and risk of complications and/or morbidity or mortality of patient management). To qualify for a particular level of MDM, two of the three elements for that level of MDM must be met or exceeded. See Table 2: Levels of Medical Decision Making (MDM) on the following page.◀	New	
▶**Table 2 Levels of Medical Decision Making (MDM)**◀ *(For this table, see Table 3 in Chapter 2 of this book.)*	New	
▶**Time**◀	New	
▶For instructions on using time to select the level of office or other outpatient E/M services code, see the ***Time*** subsection in the ***Guidelines Common to All E/M Services.***◀	New	
Unlisted Service	Relocated	**From:** Middle of Guidelines
An E/M service may be provided that is not listed in this section of the CPT codebook. When reporting such a service, the appropriate unlisted code may be used to indicate the service, identifying it by "Special Report," as discussed in the following paragraph. The "Unlisted Services" and accompanying codes for the E/M section are as follows: **99429** **Unlisted preventive** medicine service **99499** **Unlisted evaluation and management** service	Relocated	

E/M Guideline Changes	Action	From/To (for Relocated Text)
Special Report	Relocated	**From:** Middle of the Guidelines Section
An unlisted service or one that is unusual, variable, or new may require a special report demonstrating the medical appropriateness of the service. Pertinent information should include an adequate definition or description of the nature, extent, and need for the procedure and the time, effort, and equipment necessary to provide the service. Additional items that may be included are complexity of symptoms, final diagnosis, pertinent physical findings, diagnostic and therapeutic procedures, concurrent problems, and follow-up care.	Relocated	
Clinical Examples	Relocated	**From:** Middle of the Guidelines Section
Clinical examples of the codes for E/M services are provided to assist in understanding the meaning of the descriptors and selecting the correct code. The clinical examples are listed in Appendix C. Each example was developed by the specialties shown.	Relocated	
The same problem, when seen by different specialties, may involve different amounts of work. Therefore, the appropriate level of encounter should be reported using the descriptors rather than the examples.	Relocated	

APPENDIX B

Online Resources and Other Related Materials

The following are additional AMA resources that are pertinent to the CPT E/M 2021 changes. In addition, see the additional online resources that may be of use and/or interest in furthering your knowledge and perspective of the 2021 E/M changes.

For your EHR, billing system needs, coding needs, training needs, etc, check out the following American Medical Association's (AMA's) publications, services, and CPT 2021 E/M office visit coding-decision support tools and mobile app:

- E/M Office Visit Compendium 2021 Data File provides the following content and more:
  - Presentations: video and audio clips and Power Point® slides from experts
  - *CPT® Assistant articles*
  - Knowledge Base Q&A and clinical examples
  - Tables and figures
- CPT® E/M Office Visit Coder app is a modern responsive web application built using the latest technologies. It is an interactive E/M calculator tool (web application) that is designed to embed within your software as an educational and informational resource for your clinical, coding and billing users. It enables users to input minimal encounter parameters and receive a recommended CPT code, or to select a CPT code and understand what encounter parameters are required for that code. An elegant UX educates users on the new E/M office & outpatient visit guidelines with official CPT content built into the workflows.
- CPT QuickRef mobile app is downloadable through iTunes or Google Play providing quick access to code information. The 2021 coding and billing pack or multi-year coding and billing pack are available for in-app purchase and include access to an E/M Wizard to quickly determine the correct code based on patient-visit parameters.
- AMA EdHub™ eLearning modules:
  - EM Office Code Revisions: Overview
  - EM Office Code Revisions: New Ways to Report Using MDM
  - EM Office Code Revisions: New Ways to Report Using Time
- AMA *CPT Changes 2021: An Insider's View* is a publication that provides all the changes for CPT 2021 and the rationales for those changes. Clinical examples for new/revised codes are provided as appropriate.
- *CPT 2021 E/M Express Reference Coding Card* is a publication in the form of a laminated card that includes the top most-reported E/M codes with E/M guidelines and tables, which serve as a quick and handy look-up and reference tool.

- *CPT Assistant Newsletter* is the official source for CPT coding guidance.
- *Clinical Example of Radiology Newsletter* is a practical guide to correct coding for radiology.
- *CPT KnowledgeBase* provides a service in which real-life questions are answered by CPT experts. It's available as an online subscription or licensed content for integration.

For additional online resources about E/M 2021 changes, see the following sites listed.

For general overview discussions about CPT E/M office visit revisions:
https://www.ama-assn.org/practice-management/cpt/cpt-evaluation-and-management

For CMS information about patients over paperwork:
https://www.cms.gov/About-CMS/Story-Page/patients-over-paperwork

For a discussion of the E/M 2021 changes in the *AAOS Now*:
https://www.aaos.org/aaosnow/2020/apr/managing/managing01/

For an article from the AAFP about preparing for E/M coding changes:
https://www.aafp.org/news/practice-professional-issues/20200528emresources.html

For information regarding E/M changes for 2021 from ACOG:
https://www.acog.org/practice-management/coding/coding-library/evaluation-and-management-changes-for-2021

For an article about the E/M coding changes for 2021 from CHEST physician:
https://www.mdedge.com/chestphysician/article/208504/society-news/coding-changes-coming-soon

For discussion about the E/M coding changes from ASCO Practice Central:
https://practice.asco.org/em-changes-coming-soon